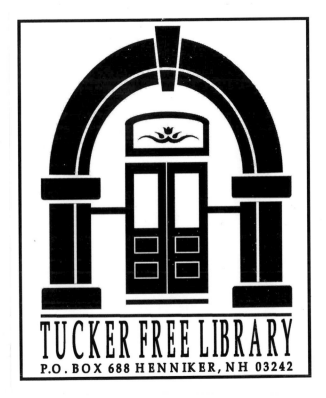

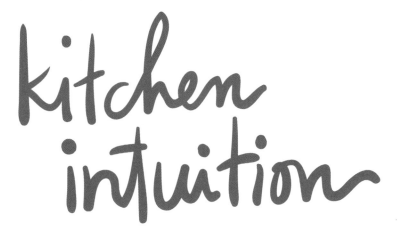

DEVYN SISSON

COOK WITH **YOUR HANDS.** **LAUGH** WITH **YOUR BELLY.**
TRUST YOUR **INTUITION.**

PRIMAL
BLUEPRINT
PUBLISHING

Kitchen Intuition: Cook with your hands. Laugh with your belly. Trust your intuition.

Mention of specific companies, organizations, or authorities in this book does not imply endorsement by the author or publisher. Information in this book was accurate at the time researched. The author received no incentives or compensation to promote the item recommendations in the book.

Library of Congress Cataloging-in-Publication Data

Names: Sisson, Devyn, 1991- author.
Title: Kitchen intuition : cook with your hands, laugh with your belly, trust
  your intuition / by Devyn Sisson.
Description: Oxnard, CA : Primal Blueprint Publishing, [2017] | Includes
  index.
Identifiers: LCCN 2017002792 (print) | LCCN 2017004145 (ebook) | ISBN
  9781939563231 (hardcover) | ISBN 9781939563378 (epub)
Subjects: LCSH: Cooking. | Creative ability in cooking. | LCGFT: Cookbooks.
Classification: LCC TX714 .S57 2017 (print) | LCC TX714 (ebook) | DDC
  641.5--dc23
LC record available at https://lccn.loc.gov/2017002792

Editor: Tracy Kearns
Design, Layout, and Hand Lettering: Caroline De Vita
Cover Design: Janée Meadows
Index and Proofreading: Tim Tate
Photography: Austin Daniels

Publisher: Primal Blueprint Publishing, 1641 S. Rose Ave., Oxnard, CA 93033
For information on quantity discounts, please call 888-774-6259 or 310-317-4414,
email: info@primalblueprintpublishing.com, or visit PrimalBlueprintPublishing.com.

DISCLAIMER: The ideas, concepts, and opinions expressed in this book are intended to be used for educational purposes only. This book is sold with the understanding that the author and publisher are not rendering medical advice of any kind, nor is this book intended to replace medical advice, nor to diagnose, prescribe, or treat any disease, condition, illness, or injury. It is imperative that before beginning any diet, exercise, or lifestyle program, including any aspect of the methodologies mentioned in *Kitchen Intuition* in general, you receive full medical clearance from a licensed physician. If you are currently taking medication for health conditions, are pregnant or a growing youth, or have a current or past condition such as cardiovascular disease, cancer, diabetes, or other serious health condition, major dietary changes should be considered with extreme caution and the guidance of a trusted medical professional. The author and publisher claim no responsibility to any person or entity for any liability, loss, or damage caused or alleged to be caused directly or indirectly as a result of the use, application, or interpretation of the material in this book. If you object to this disclaimer, you may return the book to publisher for a full refund.

Printed in the U.S.A.

Thank you, Mom and Dad,
for inspiring us all to be healthier.
I learned how to make some of my favorite (unhealthy) dishes
in a creative and nutritious way. I got to learn how to do it
on my own; to honor my preferences and pave my own way.
I am truly honored when you ask me to cook for dinner parties.

Thank you, Bro, for being a vegetarian!
You set an example and have always influenced me to
eat more green things (which are now my favorites)!
Thanks also for always sharing your vegetables in the refrigerator
and for role modeling listening to your gut.

Thank you to my friends who come over hungry,
consistently clean their plates, and bring their best SELVES
to keep me feeling encouraged and supported.
You know who you are.

Thank you to M.W. for being a notoriously picky eater,
which has challenged my creativity.
Thank you also for cooking with and for me, and
for speaking so highly of my dishes to complete strangers.

—Devyn

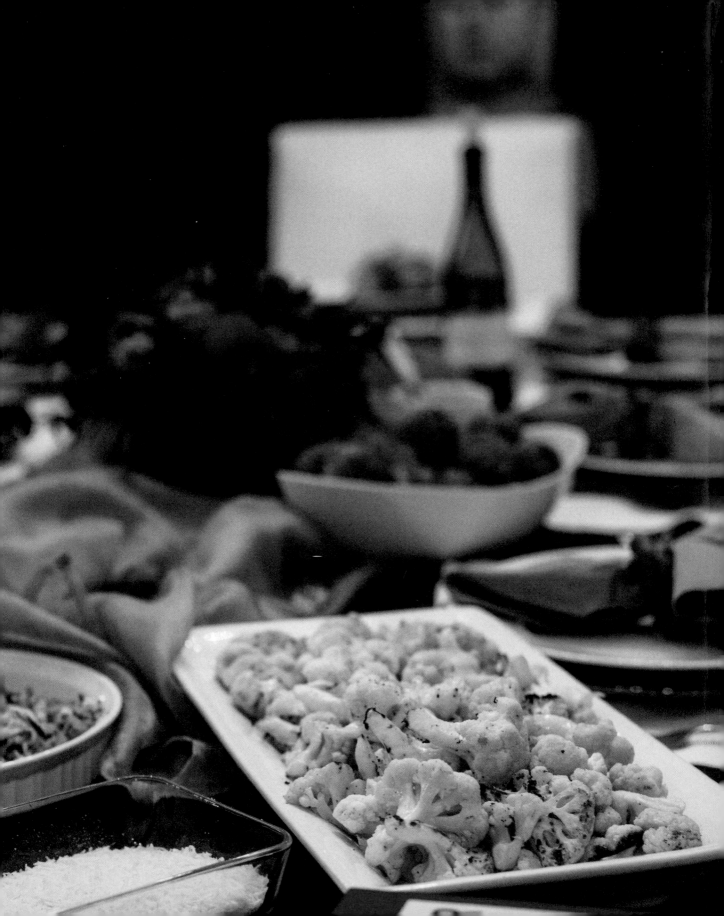

Table of Contents

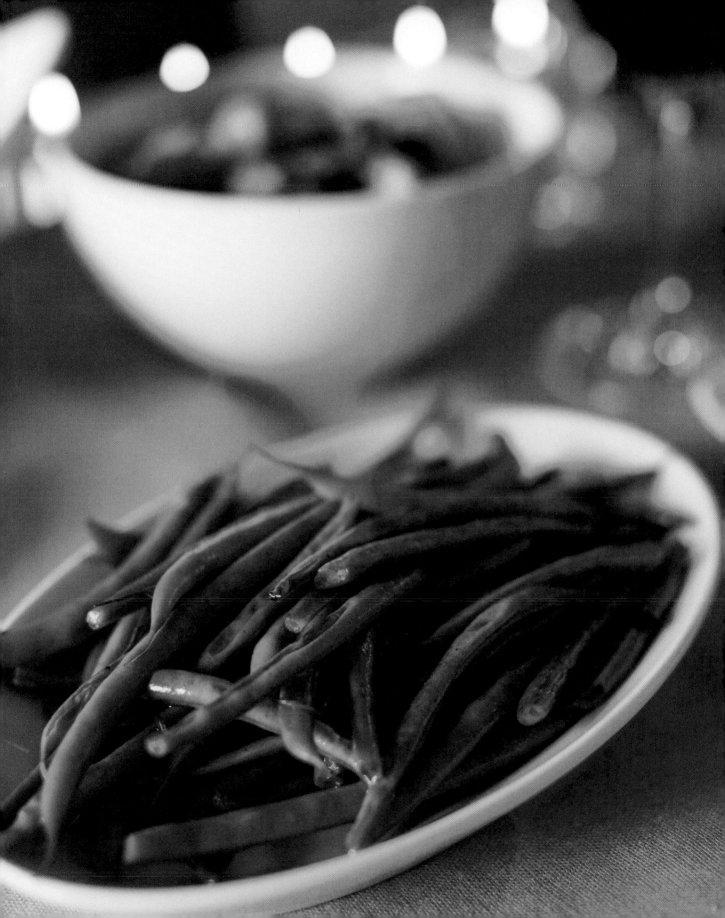

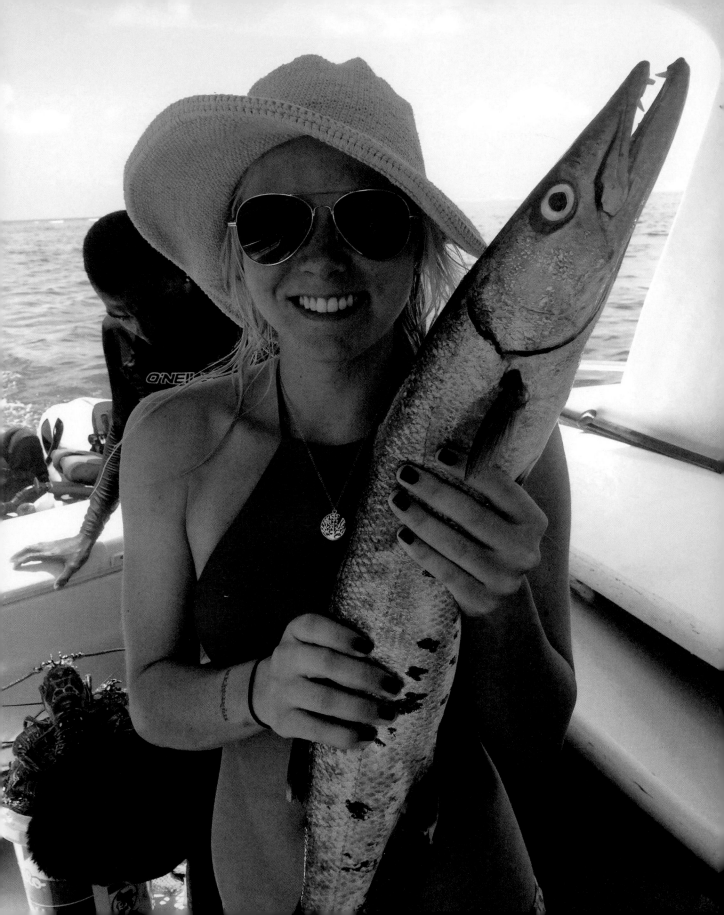

Dear Reader,

This is a book of "guessipes" or lists of ingredients I have thrown together using my intuition. It is a book of things I love to eat, cook, and share with my family and friends. If you're reading these words, I consider you a friend, and I'm excited to share with you how I am learning to nourish myself—body, mind, and spirit—and how to do so using my intuition.

I'm more interested in suggesting *how* you choose to cook, rather than *what* you choose to eat. Though filled with delicious, often primal-aligned recipes, this cookbook is really about encouraging you to become a little more conscious, a little more mindful, and a little more playful in your experience with food.

There are a million different theories on diets and lifestyles, all competing against one another, perhaps for the purpose of book sales and blog visits. Yet you might be surprised to learn how much those diverse diets have in common. According to most nutritional theories, if you can avoid processed food and sugar, limit your intake of alcohol and caffeine, and physically move your body each day, you're on the right track.

We are what we eat. This is the simplest and most overlooked concept in the medical profession—a community that has become obsessed with trying to fix problems rather than prevent them. It's no surprise that so many of us are "fat, sick, and nearly dead," as the wellness advocate, entrepreneur, and writer Joe Cross would say.

This book is a reminder to tap into your intuition, that wise inner voice that knows when, what, and how much your body needs to stay healthy and strong. All of us can access this intuition. Slow down and listen.

Taking care of your health—physical, emotional, and spiritual—means learning how to love and nourish yourself by developing a friendlier relationship with food. As with any relationship, you're probably going to stumble and make mistakes. You might add too much salt to a dish, or mix flavors that don't really work together. That's okay. Making mistakes is an important part of the journey. Discovering that you can recover and move forward from your mistakes is what builds confidence, both in and outside the kitchen.

Enjoy the "guessipes" in my cookbook, but most importantly, have fun experimenting with your own kitchen intuition.

Love,

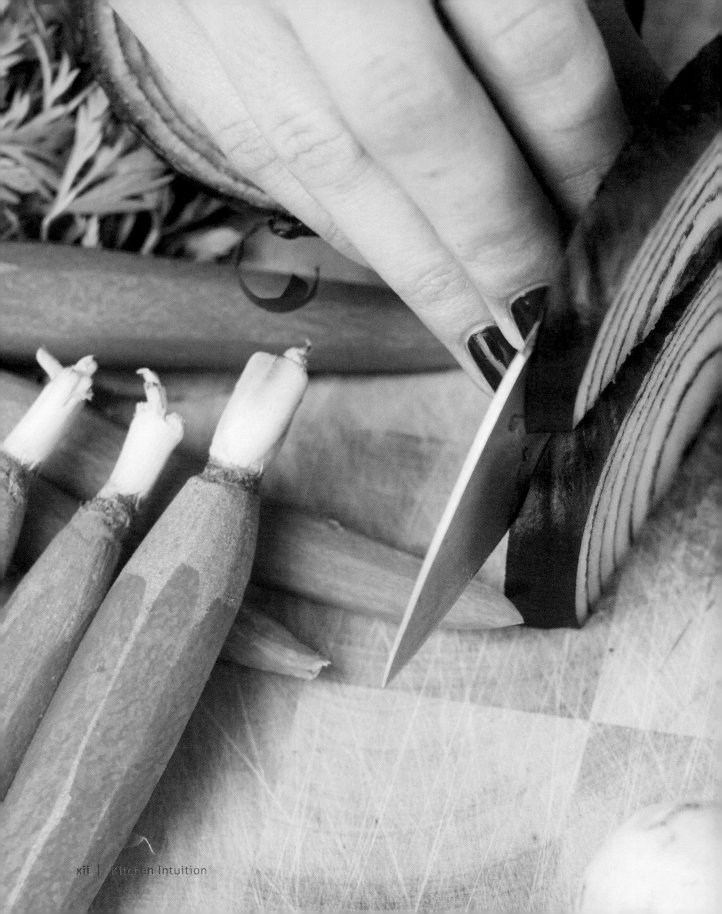

kitchen intuition

Kitchen Intuition

MAKE YOURSELF AT HOME

It certainly helps to feel comfortable while you are cooking, in as many ways as possible. Recently I discovered how much more enjoyable cooking becomes when I know where things are kept. This past winter, while vacationing in Colorado with my family, my brother and I opted to cook at home rather than go out to dinner. We decided this would be a healthier, and more interesting, dining experience. But it became quite a struggle to figure out where everything was organized in the house where we were staying. Looking around for tools while trying to cook made the experience far less fun and taught me an important lesson. Become friends with your kitchen, keep it relatively clean, and organize it in a way that makes sense. (Although sometimes organized chaos is fine, too.) It can be an adventure to cook in a new kitchen; just be aware what supplies and ingredients you have available to you BEFORE you start cooking.

Working in a strange kitchen showed me the importance of organizing utensils and spices, especially those you use most often, in easy-to-reach places. It is also useful to keep a running grocery list handy, rather than hope you'll remember to restock the ingredients you use up while cooking. Organizing your tools and keeping lists to restock takes some of the guesswork out of cooking and increases the likelihood that you will cook more often.

YOUR HANDS, YOUR TOOLS

Though I don't recommend scrambling an omelet with your fingers, your hands make great measuring tools. Use a pinch of your fingers for spices, and the palm of your hand for measuring chopped vegetables or large items for a dish. It is possible to cook an entire meal using just your hands and a knife or spatula! Believe it or not, your wrist is the best "tool" for drizzling olive oil or tossing herbs on a salad. It turns out that a kitchen fully stocked with gadgets is not nearly as important as your creativity and intuition when making delicious meals that nourish both your body and your relationships with loved ones.

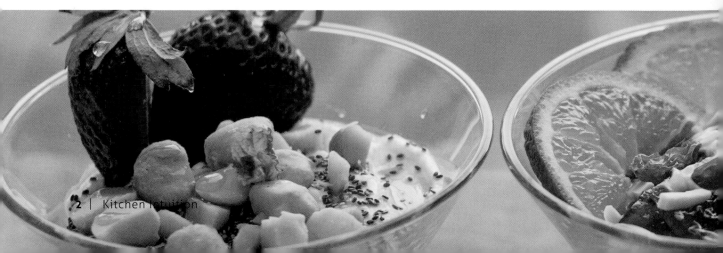

EAT ORGANIC AND LOCALLY GROWN FOOD WHEN POSSIBLE

When your budget allows, eat organic and locally grown food. The goal is to be mindful, not only of what is put into our bodies, but of what we put into the earth when producing our food. Vegetables are certainly better than processed food, but organic and/or locally grown vegetables are the best for both our health and the environment. What could be more intuitive?

Not only does shopping at your local farmers' market encourage sustainable farming and support your local growers, but buying locally grown food and planning meals around what is in season at your local market reduces the carbon footprint of your food by reducing the distance it travels to your refrigerator. Reducing the travel time of your food also increases its freshness and nutrient-value. We are all about the nutrients.

Clearly, it isn't always possible to find ingredients for a recipe that are all organic, in season, or sold at your farmers' market. Sometimes you just have to shop for veggies and meat where and when you can get them. And that's fine too. If this is the case, there are actually foods that are better choices when buying non-organic. For a general list of the most- to least-contaminated produce, I recommend the following website: www.organic.org.

MAKE IT LOOK YUMMY

We eat with our eyes first, so it is understandable that gray broccoli looks nowhere near as appetizing as a plateful of vibrant orange, roasted butternut squash with bright red cranberries and a handful of green cilantro. Can you picture it now? Getting your food to *look* good, is the first step to coaxing yourself and others to eat something that is also genuinely good for us. When I say make your food "look good," I don't mean plate the dish like it is from a Michelin-starred restaurant. You don't need to arrange your sauces on the plate to resemble a famous painting. I simply mean bring out the color. Vegetables should be bright, and cooking should enhance the color and flavor of the food, not destroy it.

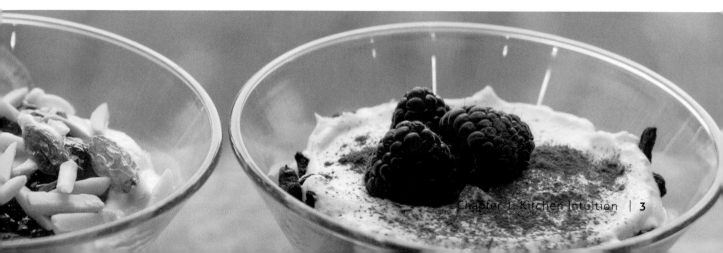

SEASON TO YOUR TASTE

Salt and pepper are your friends. Season your vegetables the way *you* like them, experimenting with any herbs and spices that you most enjoy to enhance the flavor and color of the foods you prepare. Whether following one of my recipes or not, first read through the list of ingredients and substitute in ones that suit your individual taste. I am all for trying new flavors. For instance, I encourage you to try sun-dried tomatoes and goat cheese with asparagus, unless you are not a fan of goat cheese, in which case, don't skip the recipe altogether, just try a different kind of cheese!

CUTTING THINGS

You can chop, dice, slice, mince, or CUT anything however you like. I refrain from using the "proper" cooking terms, not simply because it's a little more advanced, but frankly, it doesn't matter how the heck you cut things if you aren't working professionally in a restaurant. Be careful while you're cutting, but otherwise, cut it however you want to eat it!

When you're deciding what to cook, think about what you're making and how you want to eat it. If you're "cheffing" up some guacamole, then you probably don't want chunks of onions the size of grapes; you may want to cut them more like the size of raisins. But if you're making a salad, you don't want to cut things so small that you need a spoon to eat your veggies. Think about how you want to eat a meal when you're planning and preparing it.

INTUITION

If you purchased this book, or received it as a gift, then you are probably already familiar with the term "intuition." Odds are, you're wondering what the term could possibly mean in the kitchen.

Complements of Google:
> *Intuition:* a thing that one knows or considers likely from instinctive feeling, rather than conscious reasoning; the ability to understand something immediately, without the need for conscious reasoning.

At first thought, cooking may seem unrelated to using one's intuition. After all, we are given recipes with exact ingredients, measurements, tools, temperatures, and cooking times. On the other hand, cooking is also an art as well as a science and requires an ambiguous trusting of your gut. Sounds like a dangerous combination, right? And sometimes it is. I have totally messed up in the kitchen multiple times. Whether I strictly followed a recipe or not, things have not always turned out as hoped. And that's OK. It was all the burnt waffles, over-dressed salads, overcooked meats, and salty vegetables that have gotten me where I am today: learning to trust my gut in the kitchen.

GIVE YOURSELF PERMISSION TO MESS UP

Commit to the process, detach from the outcome.

This saying can apply to all areas of life, but we are going to use it for the kitchen. I encourage you to commit to the actual process of cooking while detaching yourself from the result. In other words, set out to enjoy the cooking AND the food, instead of being attached to making the perfect dish right off the bat. I have cooked these recipes many times, and I still find myself laughing as I hope and pray that my sautéed green beans won't be overcooked. ("Relax Dev, you'll survive.")

The difference now is that I have given myself permission to mess up, EVEN AFTER cooking something a hundred times. I don't mess up that often anymore, but it happens, especially when I am making something new! "Oh well," I tell myself, "better luck next time." Plus, I usually learn something new in the process. If you give yourself permission to mess up, it takes the pressure off and makes messing up no big deal. If you are committed to making the dish perfectly, then messing up tends to feel discouraging, making it less likely for you to try again the next night. Make sense?

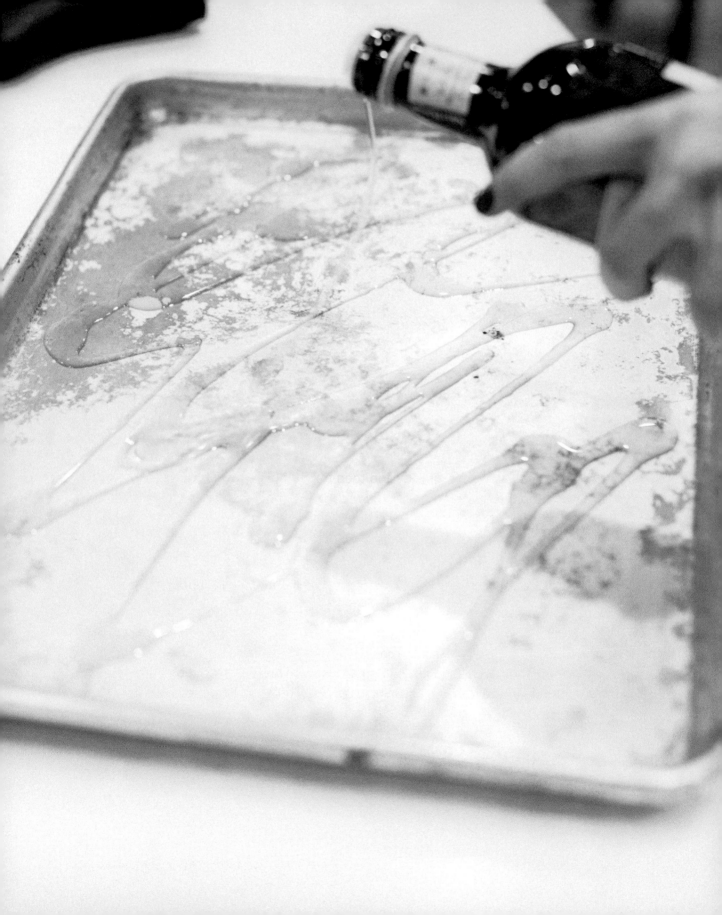

Cooking Terms: A Glossary

When you're not super-experienced in the kitchen, following a recipe can feel like tricky business. The instructions often contain terms that seem unfamiliar or irrelevant once you're standing at the counter, organic vegetables in hand. How are dicing and mincing different from one another? So I thought it might be helpful to include a list of common cooking terms with definitions that actually describe what you'll be doing.

MINCE
This usually applies to herbs, garlic, ginger or shallots,
and it means you should chop them up into teeny-tiny pieces.

CHOP
In this case you're going for pieces that are slightly smaller than bite size.

BLANCH
Boil it in hot water really quickly and then toss it into a bowl of ice water
to stop the cooking process. If we're talking about vegetables,
the color should be bright and beautiful.

ROAST
Turn on the oven and throw it on a baking sheet and bake until
it turns golden brown!

SAUTÉ
Throw whatever you've got into a hot pan with butter, coconut oil,
or olive oil and cook it until your intuition tells you its done.

FRY
Cook whatever it is in an even hotter pan with a little bit more oil
until your intuition tells you its done.

Intuitive Measurements

Cooking intuitively and to your own taste means having the courage to experiment.

When in doubt, start with less, do a taste test, and add more if desired.

Metric Conversions for Cooking

TEMPERATURE

To convert from Fahrenheit to Celsius, the formula is: $°C = (°F–32) ÷ 1.8$

Example: convert 350° F to Celsius:

$°C = (350–32) ÷ 1.8$

$°C = 318 ÷ 1.8$

$177° C$

To convert from Celsius to Fahrenheit, the formula is: $°F = (°Cx1.8) + 32$

Example: convert 200° C to Fahrenheit:

$°F = (200x1.8) + 32$

$°F = 360 + 32$

$392° F$

VOLUME

Imperial or U.S. to Metric

1 cup = 250 mL

½ cup = 125 mL

¼ cup = 60 mL

1 tablespoon = 15 mL

½ tablespoon = 8 mL

1 teaspoon = 5 mL

½ teaspoon = 2.5 mL

¼ teaspoon = 1 mL

⅛ teaspoon = .5 mL

WEIGHT

Imperial or U.S. to Metric

1 ounce = 30 grams

6 ounces = 170 grams

8 ounces (½ pound) = 225 grams

16 ounces (1 pound) = 450 grams

1 ½ pounds = 670 grams

BAKING PANS

Imperial or U.S. to Metric

5 x 9-inch loaf pan = 2 L loaf pan

9 x 13-inch cake pan = 4 L cake pan

11 x 17-inch baking sheet = 30 x 45-cm baking sheet

Wooden Spoon

Whisk

Saucepan

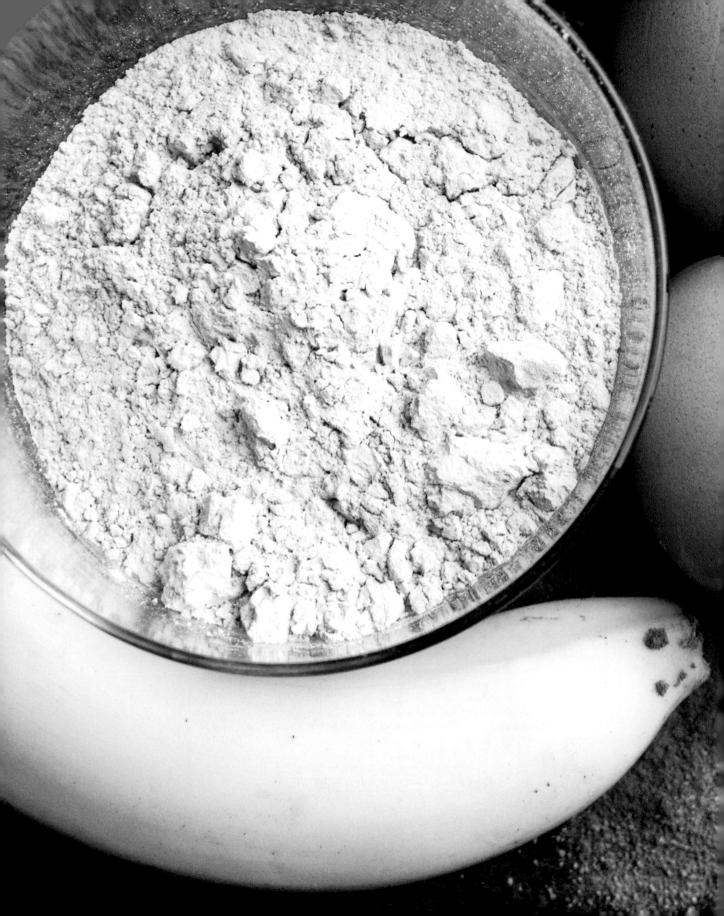

CHAPTER 2

Breakfast

"*Most of my recipes are for one to two people. Double and triple the recipe ingredients to cook for a larger group or to make enough for leftovers.*"

Kitchen Story: The Courage to Cook

It takes courage to cook, especially for others, because we all have different tastes and preferences. How could any one recipe work for all of us? After all, even a simple dish like meatloaf can be made so many different ways. This is why *Kitchen Intuition* is designed to be more of a guide with ideas for experimenting with some fun flavors, colors, and textures.

Cooking can be frustrating. You may over-salt a dish or even burn it, but the truth is, mistakes drive innovation. So have the courage to keep trying. Making a dish too bitter, sweet, or salty is part of learning how some ingredients work together (or not). Learning to cook is both an art and a science and begins when you closely check your food as you cook, tasting it when safe to do so, and making adjustments accordingly. Does it need more of a particular spice or an acidic tweak? Do you prefer more of a particular ingredient than a recipe calls for? Go ahead and add in a little more. What about the texture? Does the dish need a bit more crunch? Be sure to engage your senses. Watch as an ingredient's color, texture and smell changes during the cooking process. Sound can even assist you—sometimes popping noises suggest the temperature needs adjusting or that it is time to remove a dish from the heat altogether. Let your taste buds as well as your other senses, your intuition, and your personal preference guide you.

My recipes don't always include exact measurements—on purpose. My goal is to encourage you to work from a basic idea of approximate amounts and proportions and then to encourage you to use your nose, taste buds, and hands to make a dish your own.

If this were a baking cookbook, I'd have to be more specific about measurements as required by that type of precise cooking. But for the soups, salads, sides, and other dishes I present in *Kitchen Intuition*, there is more wiggle room to experiment and to let your intuition run wild.

By definition, intuition is to know something instinctually—without conscious reasoning. While I'll provide approximate amounts and proportions as well as cooking times, I encourage you to access your senses to help determine if something is fully cooked to *your* satisfaction. Many people start out following recipes precisely and then alter them over time to suit individual tastes. The recipes in *Kitchen Intuition* are by nature easy to prepare because they utilize familiar whole foods, spices, and herbs for the dishes and sauces.

Most of the recipes in *Kitchen Intuition* are for one to two people. By all means, double and triple the recipe ingredients to cook for a larger group or to make enough for leftovers. I have shared all of these recipes with my closest friends and family, but I have also enjoyed them on my own. Have fun making these recipes your own.

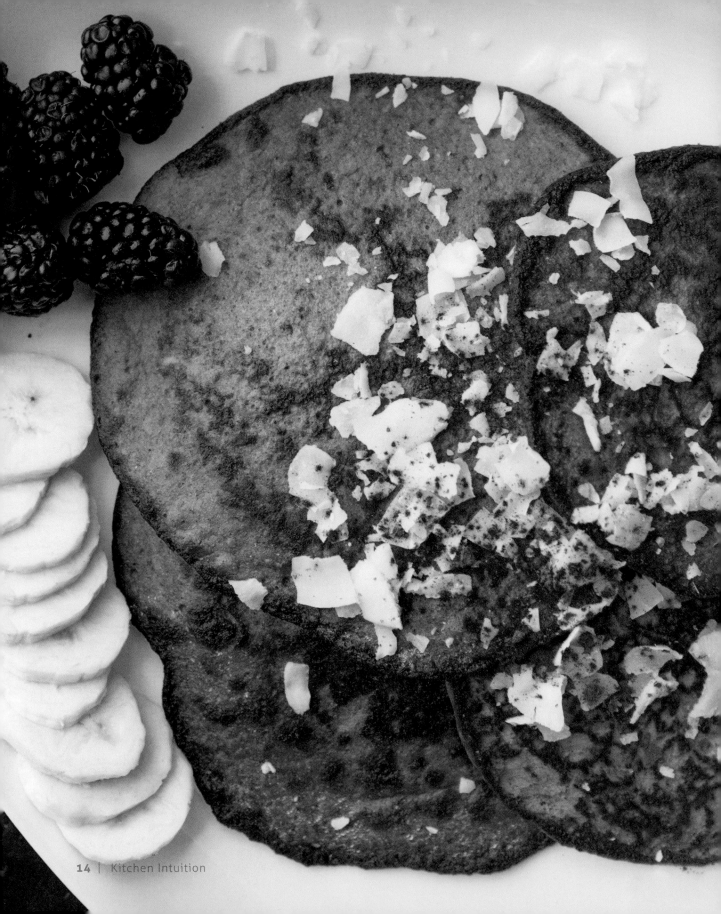

Protein Powder Pancakes

SERVES: 1

INGREDIENTS

1 banana (per pancake)

1 egg (per pancake)

1 scoop of a chocolate- or vanilla-flavored protein powder

Water (as needed)

Dash of cinnamon

Dash of nutmeg

1 tablespoon of coconut oil

Optional: berries, coconut flakes, maple syrup

METHOD

In a medium bowl, whisk one egg, and use a fork to mash up half a banana. Toss a scoop of protein powder into the bowl, adding water as needed. The consistency should be like normal pancake batter—not too runny, nor too thick. Add a dash of cinnamon and a dash of nutmeg. (I love both these spices, so I add a FEW dashes!)

Preheat a pan with some coconut oil over medium-high heat. Pour the batter into whatever shape or squiggle you choose. Cook for about 3 minutes on each side or until ready. Slice the other half of the banana and use as a topping, along with any other toppings you might enjoy such as berries, coconut flakes, or maple syrup.

GREEK
yogurt cups

SERVES: 1

You can make these yogurt cups any way you like. Find a color combo and flavors that you most like. I suggest choosing a nut or seed, berries or a dried fruit, and a flake of some sort (for a crunchy texture) mixed with sweet and sour flavors. Layer it up in a bowl and dig in!

INGREDIENTS

1 cup Greek yogurt

Small handful of nuts

Small handful of dried fruit

Small handful of seeds

Pinch or two of coconut flakes

Small handful of fresh berries

Drizzle of honey, maple syrup, or marmalade

SUGGESTIONS

Dried fruit: raisins, cranberries, dried mango or apricots

Seeds: chia or hemp seeds

Nuts: macadamia, almonds, pecans, or walnuts

SWEET TIP

To sweeten the yogurt, drizzle agave, honey, or maple syrup on the top, or mix it in a bowl before you begin to assemble the yogurt cup. My advice... get creative.

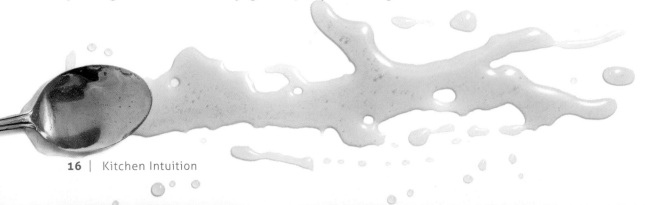

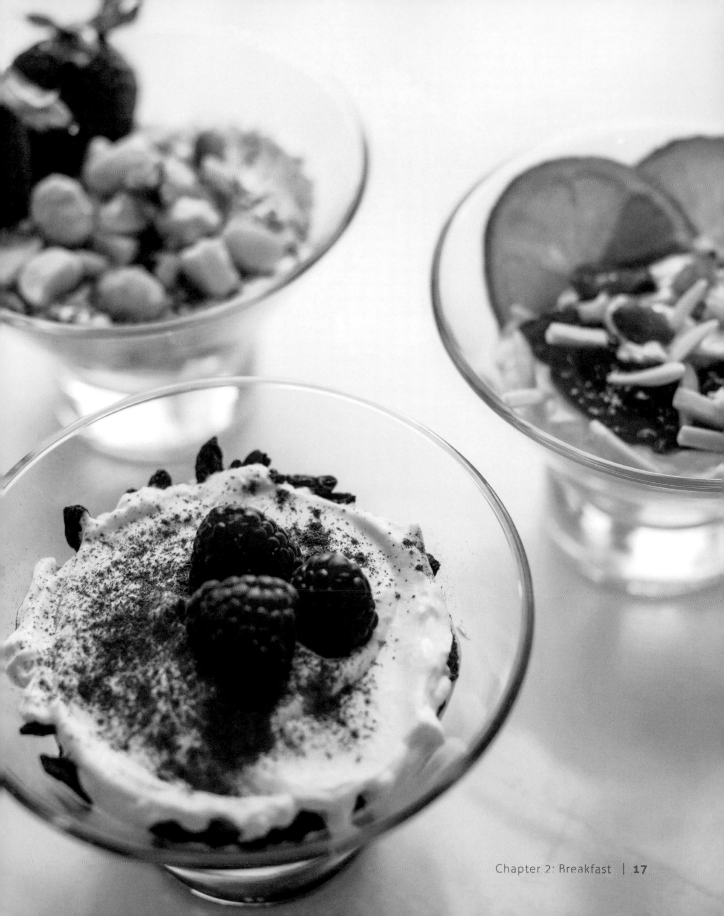

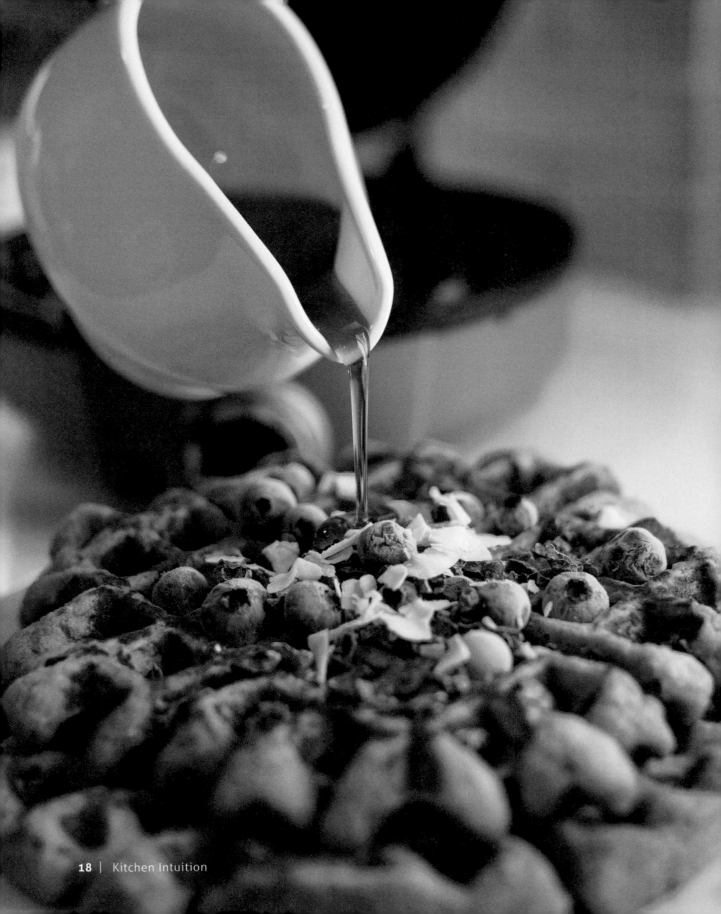

THE BEST
Banana Almond Flour Waffles
SERVES: 1 TO 2 PEOPLE

There are a lot of things I choose not to eat simply because they are too processed or just don't feel good in my body. So when I discovered that I could eat waffles and feel great, I was ecstatic. When I finally figured out how to make healthy waffles, I ate them every day for weeks. (By healthy, I mean they aren't filled with processed ingredients I can't pronounce.) This recipe took some time to finagle, but I experimented and finally got the proportions down. Here's how I do it for two waffles or one big waffle, depending on the waffle iron.

INGREDIENTS

2 unripe bananas (green at the top, but not the whole thing)

2 eggs

Handful of almond meal (about ¼ to ½ cup)

NOTE: The amount of almond flour will vary depending on the size of the egg and banana. The batter should be thick, rather than runny.

METHOD

In a large bowl mash the bananas with a fork, potato masher, or my personal favorite, your hands! Add the eggs and almond meal to the bowl; mix together. Pour the batter into a preheated waffle iron and follow the waffle iron instructions for cooking.

SUGGESTIONS

These waffles are fantastic with maple syrup, berries, coconut flakes, cacao nibs, more cinnamon, almond butter, coconut cream, or ALL of the above. Go crazy and figure out how you like your waffles.

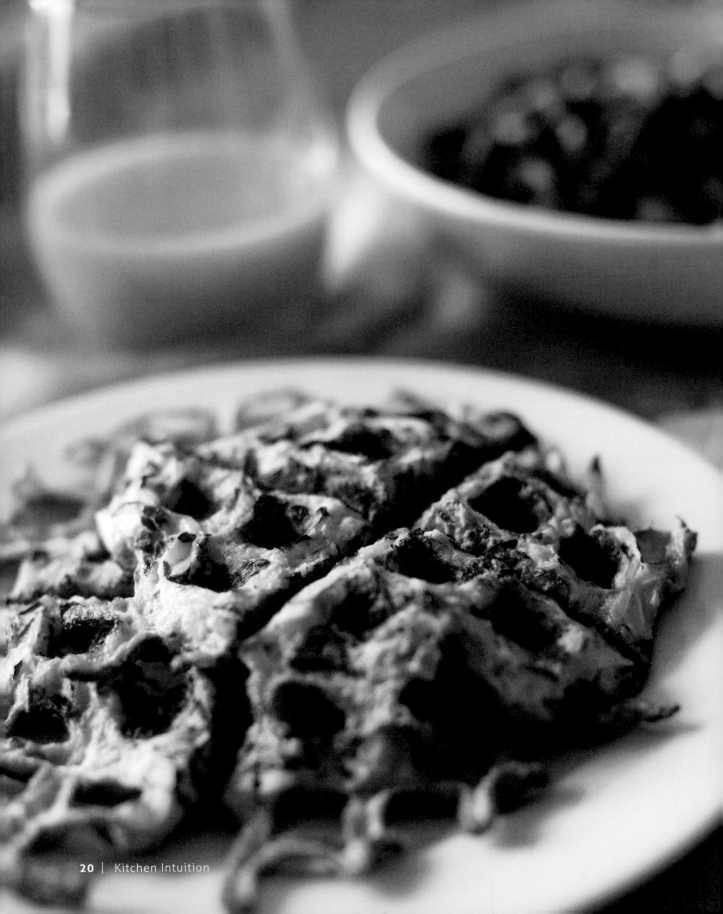

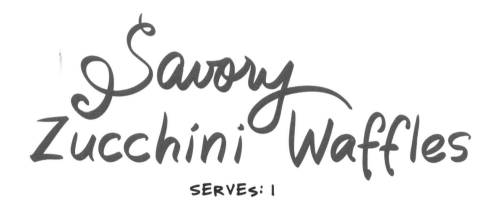

Savory Zucchini Waffles

SERVES: 1

My mom loves syrup (using any excuse to have some), so she puts maple on these bad boys. I am more a lover of savory flavors, so I usually eat these with guacamole or hummus! I've even used these waffles as bread for a breakfast sandwich. YUM!

INGREDIENTS

Zucchini (1 per waffle, depending on size)

Egg (1 per waffle)

Pinch of salt

Pinch of any herb or spice you prefer
(although, you might want to try dried basil, parsley, or thyme)

METHOD

Using a cheese grater, grate the zucchini on a paper towel or cloth. Squeeze out as much moisture out of the grated zucchini as you can. In a bowl, mix the grated zucchini with the egg and spices. Pour the waffle mix into a preheated waffle iron and cook according to your waffle iron's instructions.

VEGGIE EGG
Breakfast Muffins

MAKES: 6 EGG MUFFINS

You can put pretty much anything you want in these muffins: leftover vegetables, farmers' market finds, and meat or cheese.

INGREDIENTS

A few strips of bacon (depending on your preference)

1 to 2 zucchini, grated

1 cup of sliced mushrooms

Half an onion, diced

6 eggs

2 tablespoons butter, to grease the muffin tin

Substitution

You can substitute sausage for bacon.

METHOD

Preheat the oven to 350 degrees Fahrenheit. Cook the bacon in a hot pan until crispy, and then set aside to cool. Use a cheese grater to grate the zucchini onto a cloth or paper towel (so you can squeeze out all the moisture). Dice the onion and the mushrooms fairly small. When the bacon has cooled, chop it up or crumble it with your hands. Whisk the eggs in a bowl. Using your hands, grease the bottom and edges of a muffin tin with a pat of butter. Divide the eggs into six muffin tins. Sprinkle a little of each of your ingredients (onion, mushroom, crumbled bacon, and the grated zucchini) into each of the six cups. Bake for about 20 minutes or until the muffin tops look set, rather then wet or runny.

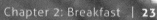

SALMON EGG WRAP

SERVES: SEVERAL PEOPLE

You can put pretty much anything you want in these wraps. I just love smoked salmon and cream cheese with all the toppings. Some days this takes the place of a bagel.

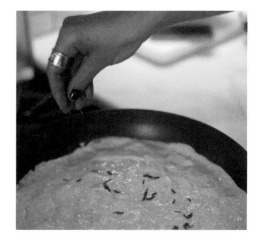

INGREDIENTS

A few eggs (about 1 per crepe)

1 package smoked salmon lox

A few sprigs of chives, chopped (or any herb you like)

Cream cheese (enough to smear on your wrap!)

Try any of the following for toppings:

¼ red onion, chopped

2 radishes, chopped

½ cucumber, sliced lengthwise

½ tomato, chopped or sliced

Spoonful of capers

1 lemon, juiced

METHOD

Heat up a good nonstick pan (really helps with the delicate eggs). Crack the eggs in a bowl and whisk them together, adding a spoonful of water. Pour a small amount of the egg into the heated pan, and swirl the pan around to spread the eggs out thin like a crepe. Add the chopped herbs. Test the egg crepe with a spatula to see if you can lift it up without breaking it. If so, give it a flip.

When the egg crepe is done and has cooled, spread a thin layer of cream cheese on it. Then add smoked salmon and any other veggies you like from the list above. Roll it up and enjoy!

FRIED EGG
Kitchen Sink Bowl

Sometimes this is a brunch item for me, but to be honest, a lot of the time it's a lazy dinner option. I pull out all the veggies I have lying around in the fridge (from dinners earlier in the week, and raw or even frozen veggies), literally everything, but the kitchen sink. I would eat this for every meal if I could. Good news, I CAN!

INGREDIENTS

1 handful of leftover vegetables

1 egg, fried

1 tablespoon of olive or coconut oil or butter

Pinch of salt (or a spice you prefer)

Small handful of arugula (or your preferred lettuce)

1 avocado (sliced)

Dash of hot sauce

METHOD

Heat the veggies quickly in a hot pan with oil or butter. Then add the veggies to a bowl of lettuce, avocado, and hot sauce. I like to throw a fried egg on top because the gooey yolk makes a delicious sauce.

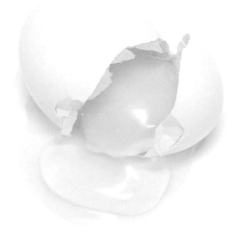

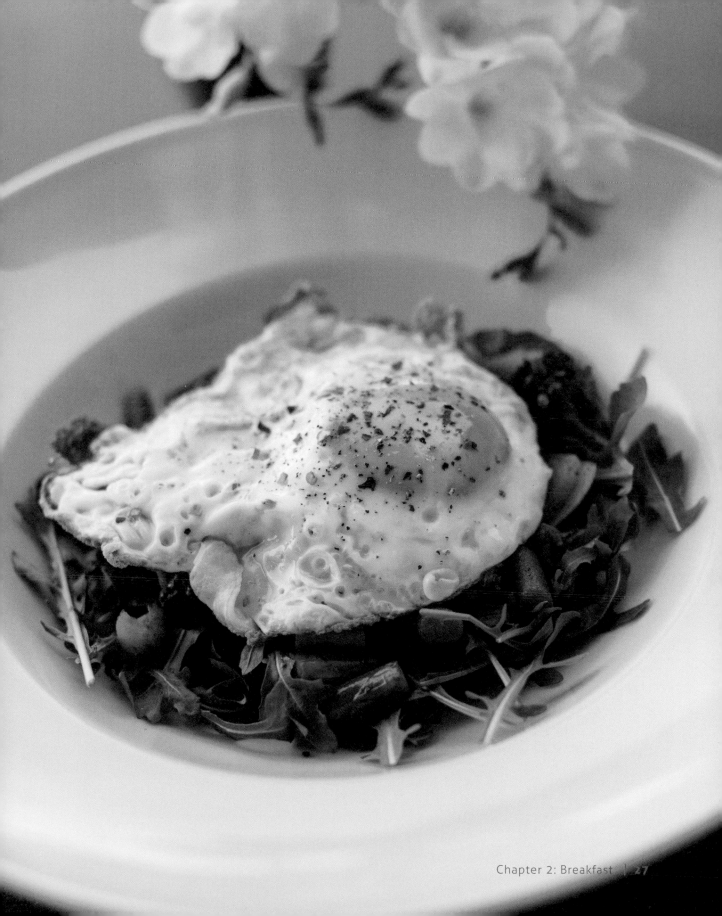

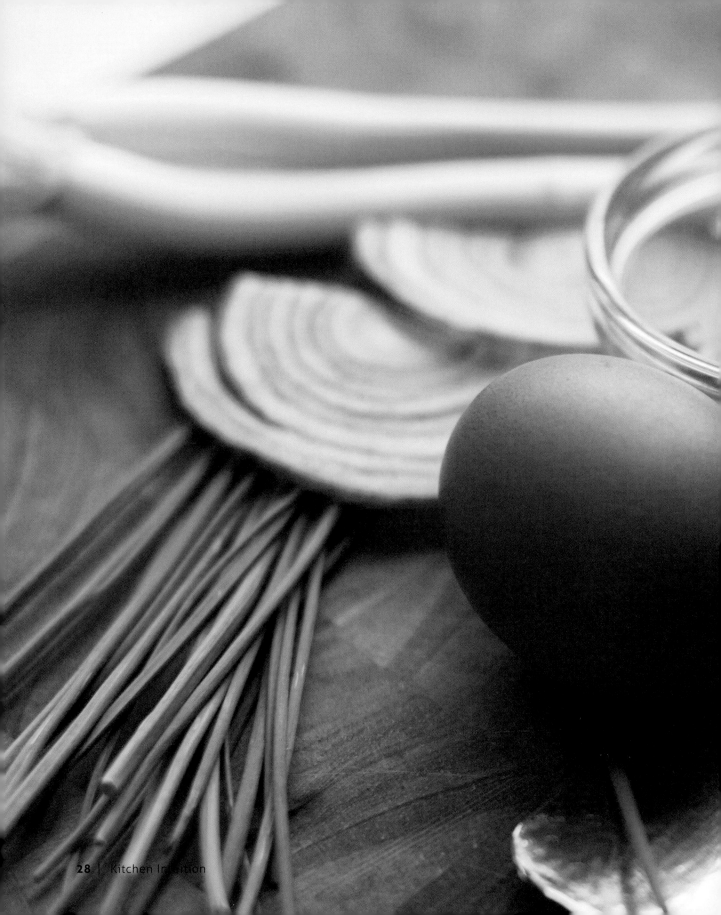

Egg (White) Crepe Sushi

Egg (white)

If you ever have people over for brunch, this is the way to go.

INGREDIENTS

8 egg whites or 1 small carton of organic egg whites

5-10 sprigs of chives (or more if you love them)

3 green onions or scallions, sliced thinly from the white to light-green part

1 package cream cheese

1-2 packages of lox (smoked salmon)

½ red onion, sliced thinly

4 radishes, sliced thinly

1 cucumber, sliced lengthwise

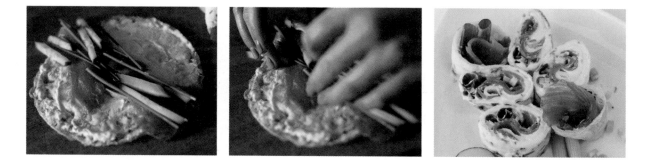

METHOD

To cook each crepe individually:

Preheat a nonstick pan (which is good for cooking delicate egg crepes). Crack an egg over a bowl, separating the egg white from the yolk. (You can also use store-bought egg whites.) Add a spoonful of water to the egg white in the bowl. Pour only a small amount of the egg white into the heated pan, and swirl the pan around to spread the egg out thin. Add the chopped chives. Test the crepe's doneness with a spatula to see if you can lift it up without breaking it. If so, give it a flip.

When the egg crepe is done and has cooled, spread a thin layer of cream cheese on it. Then add smoked salmon and any other veggies you like from the list above. Roll it up and enjoy!

Crepe Sushi

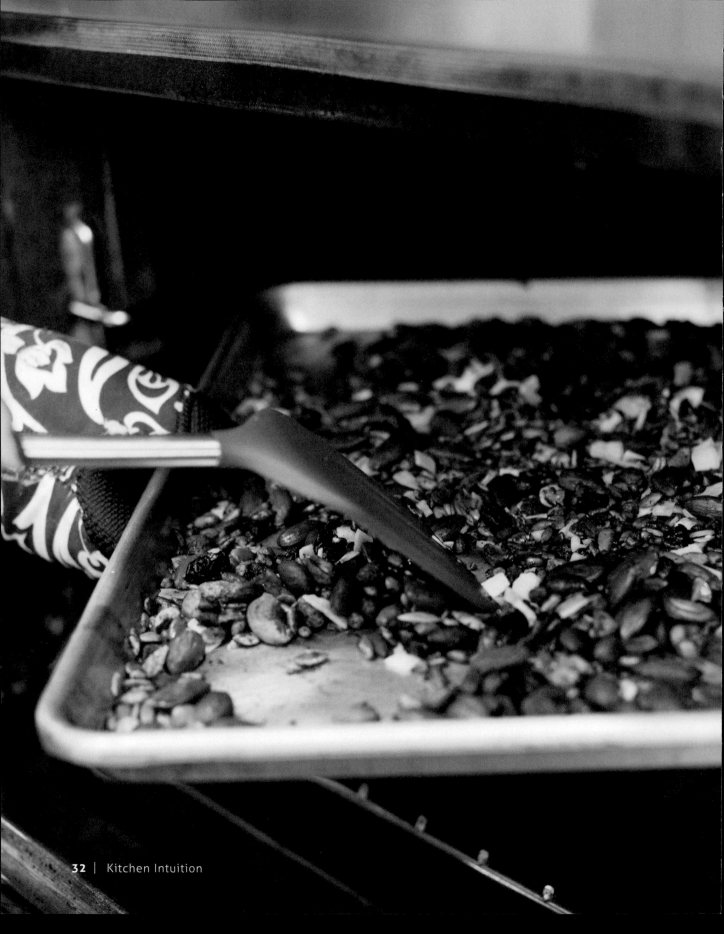

Nutty Granola

Holy moly this paleo grain-free granola is the most delicious snack/topping/cereal/breakfast/dessert ever. I usually make a big batch of this and keep it in a jar on the counter. I snack on it and add it to yogurt or coconut ice cream, or sometimes I eat the granola as cereal, throwing it in a bowl with almond or coconut milk. It has all the things I love to eat and smell packed into one delicious guessipe.

INGREDIENTS

A handful each of:

Almonds

Cashews

Walnuts

Pecans

Sunflower seeds

Pumpkin seeds

Flax seeds

Chia seeds

Small handfuls of:

Coconut flakes

Goji berries

1 to 2 tablespoons of coconut oil

A few dashes of cinnamon

2 tablespoons maple syrup

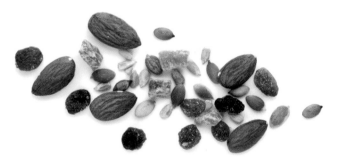

METHOD

Preheat the oven to 350 degrees Fahrenheit.

Chop the nuts slightly or leave them whole, depending on how you intend to use the granola. Combine the nuts, seeds, coconut flakes, coconut oil, maple syrup, and spices on a sheet tray, mixing the ingredients all around with your hands.

Roast the nuts for approximately 20 minutes; sometimes more, sometimes less. Just keep an eye on them and try not to burn them. (Although my dad likes the burnt batches the best.) When the nuts look golden and toasty, remove them from the oven and let cool. Add goji berries.

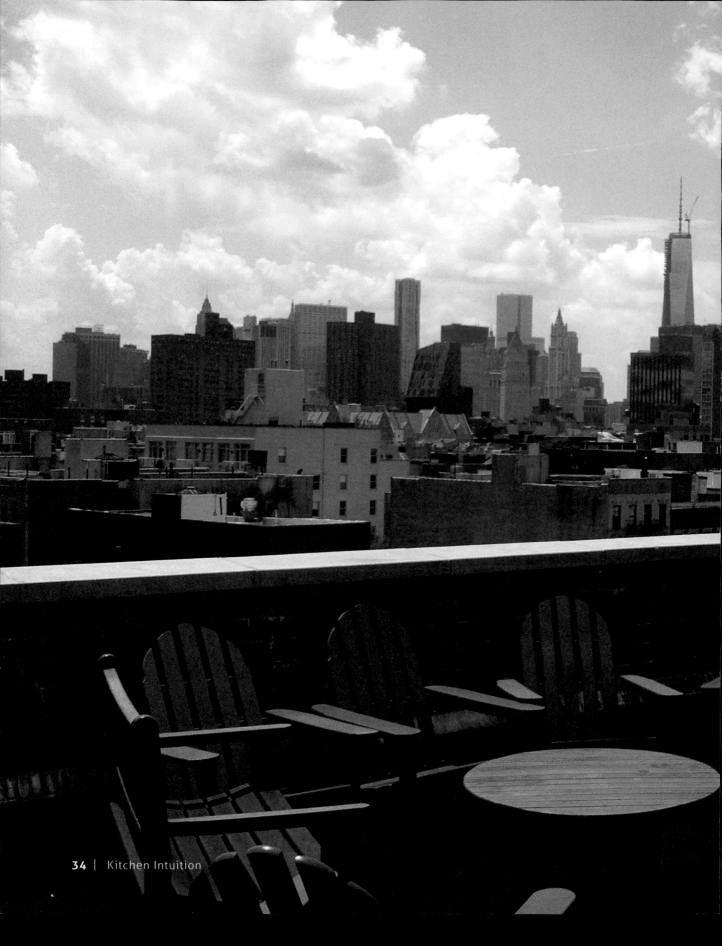

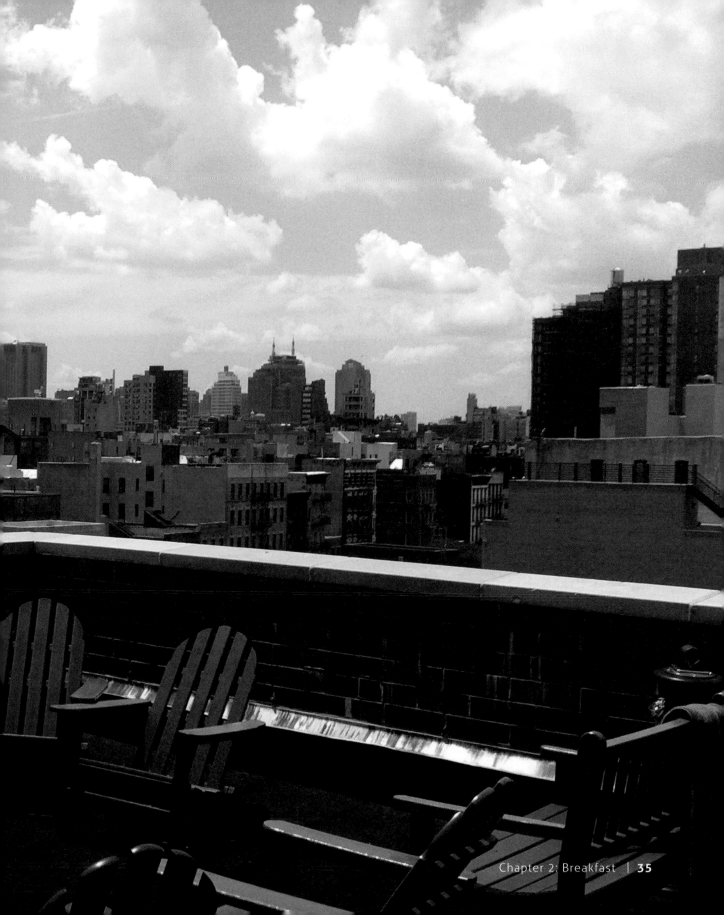

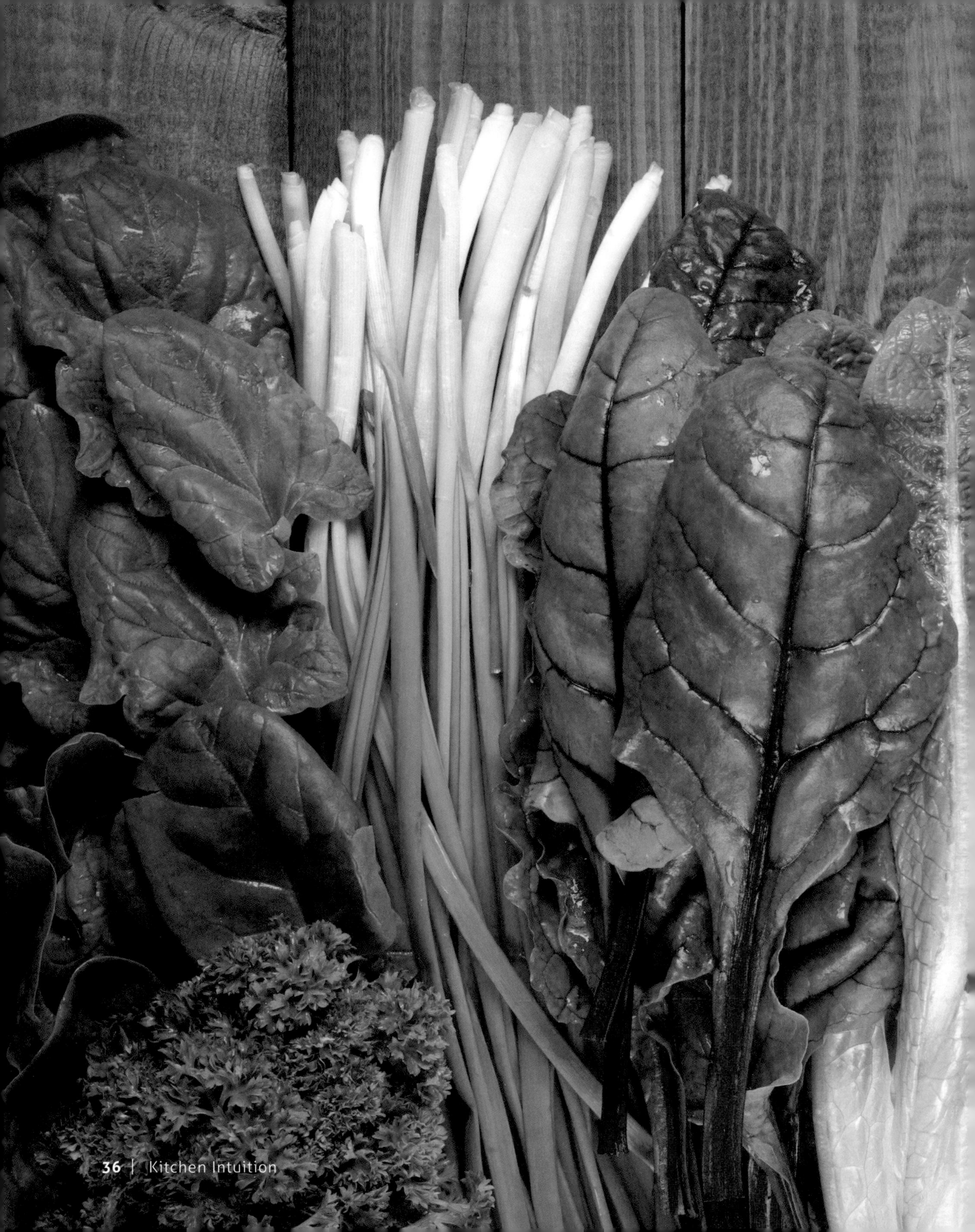

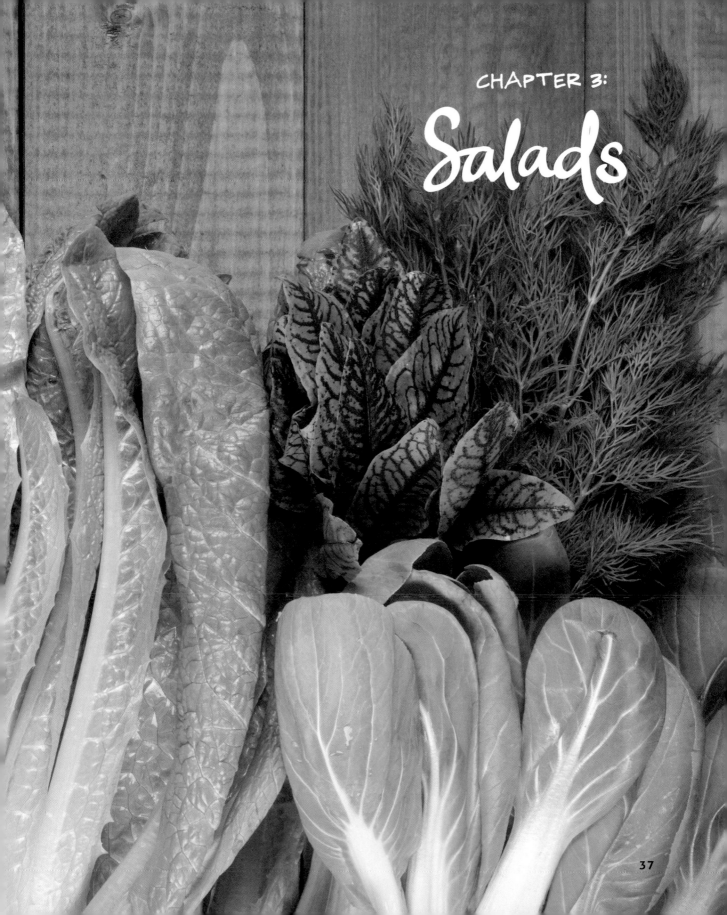

CHAPTER 3:

Salads

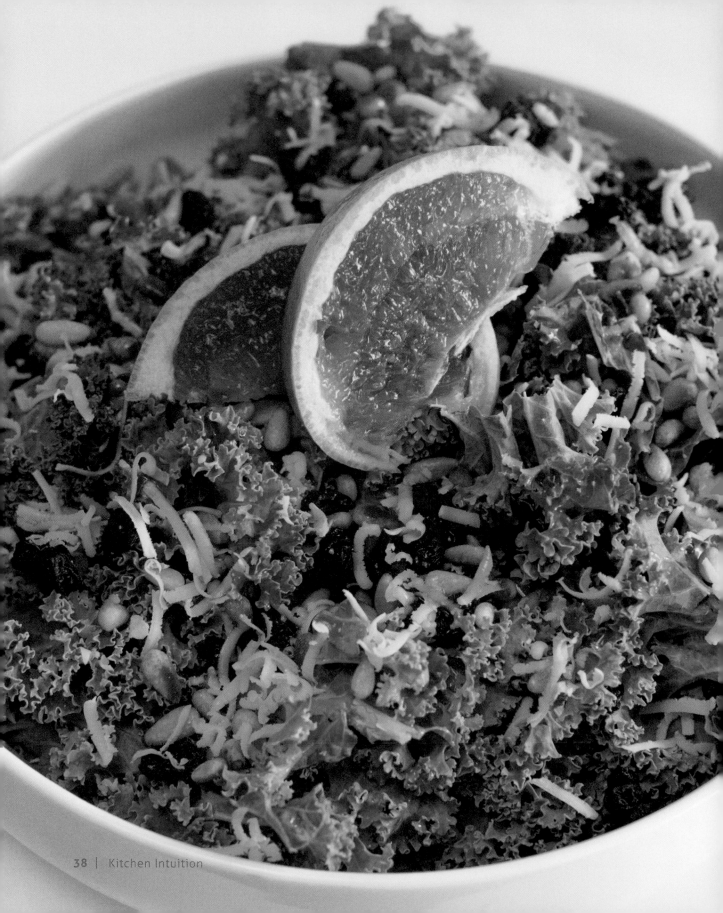

Kale Salad

SERVES: 2 TO 3 PEOPLE

I love this salad because it gets better the longer it sits. Raw kale has a chewy, crunchy texture. Parmesan provides salty goodness. Pine nuts add a soft, nutty flavor. And raisins and grapefruit juice burst in your mouth. There are so many variations of this salad. Don't hesitate to experiment on your own!

INGREDIENTS

1 bunch of kale

Small handful of pine nuts

Medium handful of Parmesan cheese, grated

Small handful of raisins

Half a medium grapefruit, juiced

Drizzle of olive oil

Pinch of salt and pepper

Substitutions

pine nuts – walnuts, slivered almonds

Parmesan – goat cheese

raisins – dried cranberries or any dried fruit

grapefruit juice – lemon or lime

METHOD

Get your (clean) hands dirty! You barely need kitchen tools for this one. Start by throwing a handful of pine nuts into a hot pan to toast them lightly and quickly. Keep an eye on them because they tend to burn easily. When toasted, set the pine nuts aside to cool. Wash the kale. Use your hands to tear up the leaves into bite-size pieces, discarding the vein that runs down the middle of the leaf.

Put the kale in a large bowl for combining ingredients. Throw in a handful of raisins, (cooled) pine nuts, and some salt and pepper to taste. Drizzle some olive oil and squeeze half a grapefruit over the salad and toss the ingredients together.

If you would like, grate and add a handful of Parmesan cheese, once again mixing everything together. Give it a taste and see what YOUR taste buds need to make it even better! Enjoy with friends or in a peaceful setting alone.

Butter Lettuce Salad

SERVES: 3 TO 4 PEOPLE

I owe the concept of this delicious salad to my friend Sydney. It is an interesting combination of ingredients that come together to form the most light, enjoyable, and satisfying summer salad.

INGREDIENTS

1 head of butter or romaine lettuce

Large handful of cherry tomatoes

½ avocado

3 to 5 stalks of hearts of palm, canned

Drizzle of olive oil

Splash of balsamic vinegar

Dollop of mustard

Pinch of salt and pepper

Small handful of slivered almonds

METHOD

Wash and tear up one head of lettuce and set in a bowl.

Slice a handful of cherry tomatoes in halves or quarters, depending on their size. Cut half of an avocado into small, bite-size pieces. Slice a few stalks of hearts of palm into bite-size pieces. Add all the veggies to the bowl with the lettuce.

In a separate bowl whisk together the olive oil, balsamic vinegar, and mustard for the salad dressing. Pour the dressing over the salad and toss. Season with salt and pepper to taste and garnish with a handful of slivered almonds. Give it a try to see what other flavors your taste buds might enjoy, and then add them.

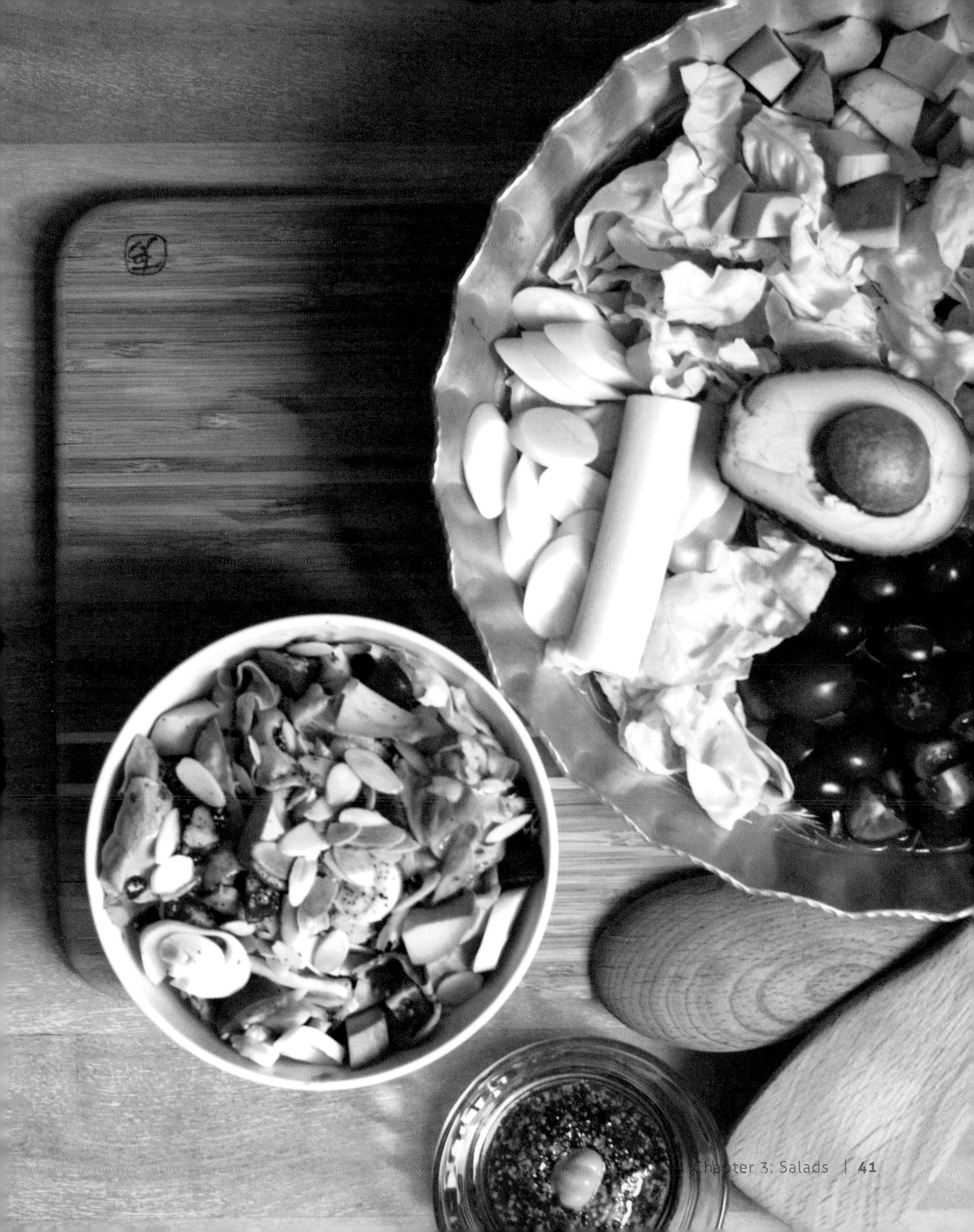

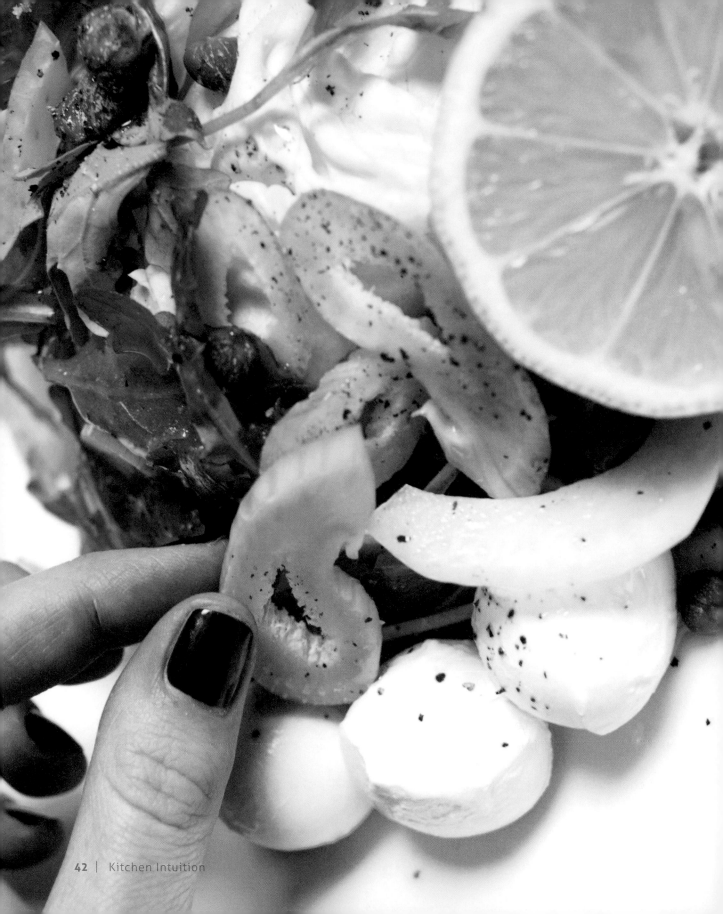

Arugula Salad

This is my favorite simple salad because I love arugula. It has such a strong flavor (for a lettuce) and it goes well with salty capers and Parmesan cheese. This is also good with bits of mozzarella and slices of tomato for a beautiful red color. I pair this salad with literally any protein, but it is especially good with tuna on top for a light lunch.

INGREDIENTS

1 head or bag of arugula

Small handful of Parmesan cheese

1 handful of capers

Drizzle of olive oil

Splash of white vinegar

Pinch of salt and pepper

Optional: tuna

Substitutions

arugula – mixed greens, red lettuce

Parmesan – burrata, mozzarella, white cheddar

capers – chopped pickles, olives

METHOD

Throw washed arugula in a bowl (no need to cut or tear).

Toss in a handful of capers or any salty, pickled thing you enjoy. Drizzle some olive oil over the top and then a quick splash of vinegar. Add a pinch of salt and pepper and shaved Parmesan (or pieces of mozzarella, burrata or cheddar cheese). Toss together and give it a taste.

Add chunks of tuna or anything else you can think of to make it even more delicious.

Quinoa Greek Salad

SERVEs: 2 OR 3 pEopLE

This is my go-to side dish for even the pickiest of eaters. I love a traditional Greek salad, but it isn't always enough. This one is a bit more filling, and it's great with a small piece of fish or chopped chicken mixed in. This salad is best cold, but sometimes I can't wait until the quinoa has cooled down to mix it all together. I like to keep the dressing light so that it doesn't get soggy, but I pack in the flavor with herbs and spices. This is a great lunch to make ahead for the next day—with or without the added protein.

INGREDIENTS

3 cups of quinoa (cooked according to the package instructions)

1 large tomato or 1 handful of cherry tomatoes

½ cucumber

½ red onion

Small handful of black olives

Small handful of chopped cilantro

½ bell pepper

Drizzle of olive oil

Splash of white vinegar

Handful of feta cheese

Pinch of chopped oregano, fresh or dried

Pinch of salt and pepper

Substitutions

quinoa – cooled, brown rice

cilantro – parsley, dill, chives

METHOD

Cook the quinoa according to the packaging instructions and set aside. Then chop a large tomato into small pieces or cut cherry tomatoes in half. Chop the half cucumber into smaller, bite-size pieces. Chop the half red onion (or the whole thing if you want to store and use later). Halve the olives, discarding the pits. Chop the half bell pepper.

Add all the veggies to the bowl of cooled quinoa (if you can wait that long). Drizzle olive oil and then splash some white vinegar over all the ingredients. Mix all the salad ingredients together, and then add the crumbled feta, oregano, and cilantro (or any herbs of your choice). Season with salt and pepper.

Give it a try. What you think? Are your taste buds calling out for any other flavors?

> ### COOKING TIP
> I usually use the other half of the pepper, onion, and tomato, and rest of the feta cheese to make a delicious omelet the next morning for breakfast.

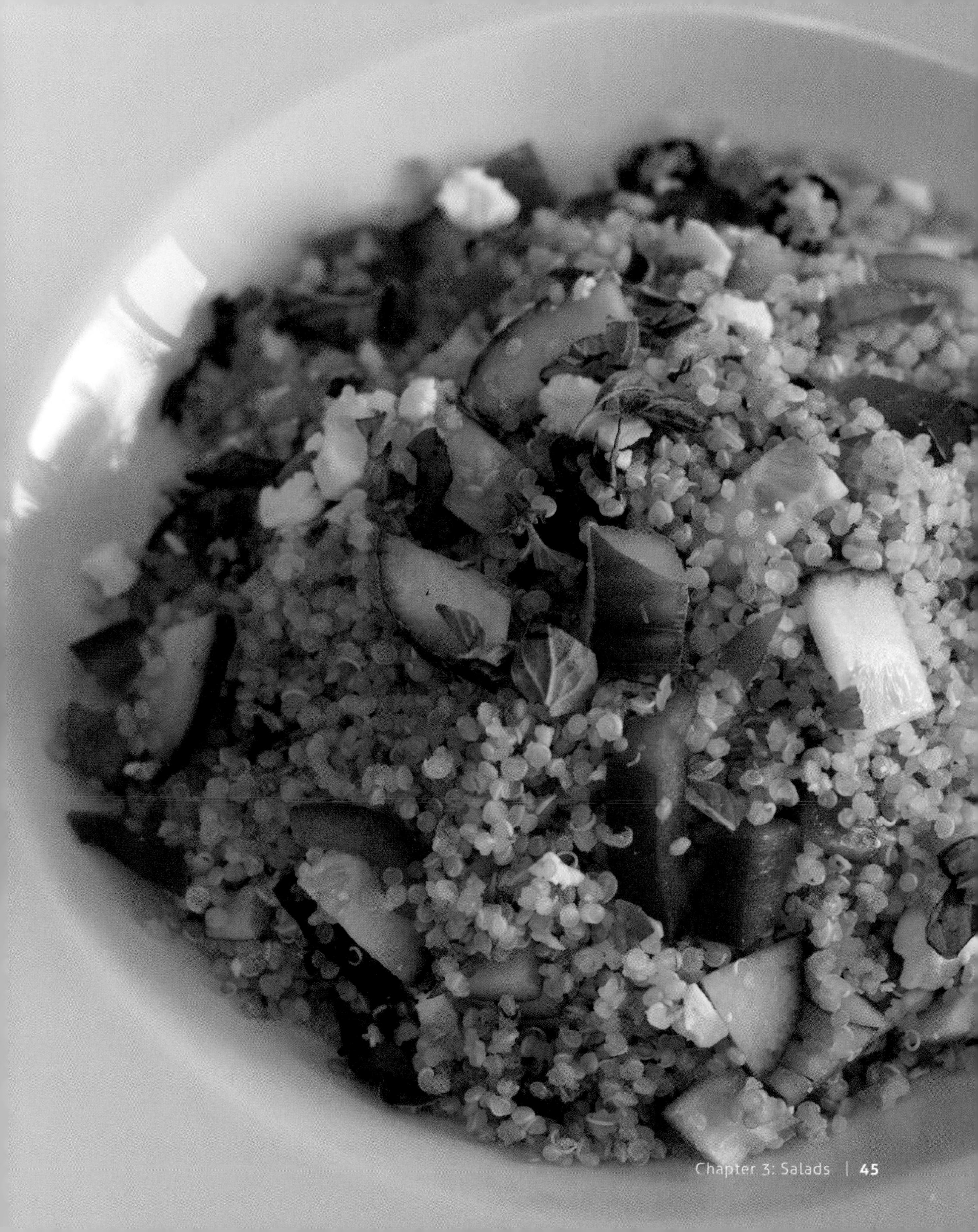

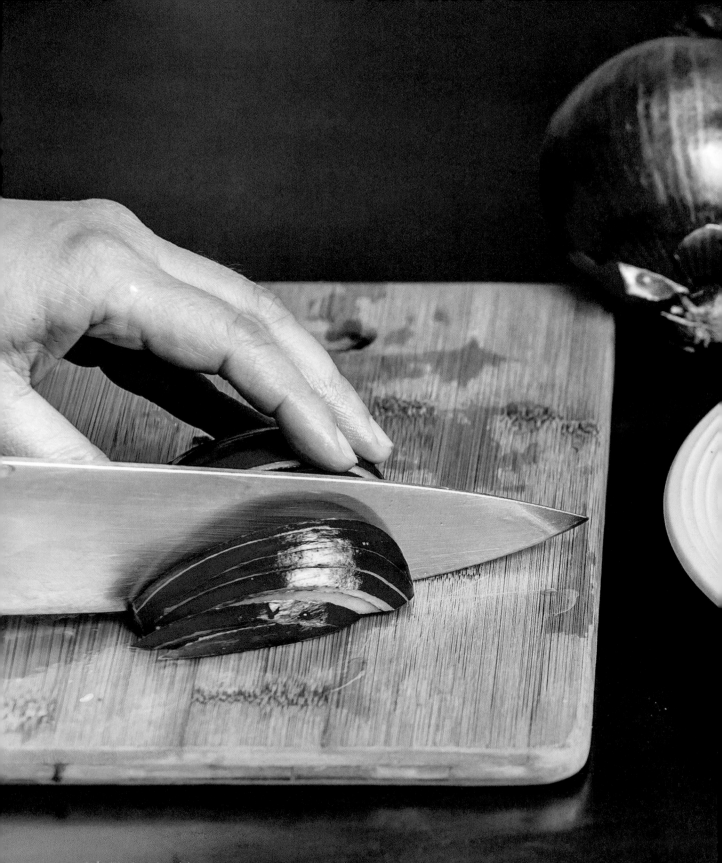

Cucumber Salad

INGREDIENTS

3 parts rice vinegar

1 part sesame oil

½ red onion

1 cucumber

A few sprigs chopped cilantro leaves

Small handful sesame seeds

Optional: pinch of sugar

METHOD

Mix together 3 parts rice vinegar and 1 part sesame oil. (You can add a TINY pinch of sugar or honey to cut some of the acid). Thinly slice the half red onion and mix into the dressing so the onion can start to marinate a bit. Cut up the cucumber in cubes or slices (however you like them), then add to the dressing. Add cilantro and sesame seeds, and mix everything together.

Give it a taste and see what you think. Sometimes I add a dash of soy sauce or some red chili flakes. Use your intuition to make it your own!

EVERYTHING
but the...
S A L A D

This is a suggested list of ingredients for a salad based on what was in my fridge and pantry when I wrote this cookbook. But you can take pretty much anything from the fridge, throw it on a bowl of lettuce, and call it a yummy salad for lunch or dinner! It is especially great for a weeknight meal when you may have a bunch of stuff in the fridge, but not a ton of time.

INGREDIENTS

Small handful of chopped tomatoes

Small handful of chopped bell peppers

Leftover veggies (roasted, grilled, or steamed)

Small handful of black beans, canned

Handful of cubed cheese (like cheddar)

Drizzle of olive oil

Splash of white vinegar

½ lemon, juiced

Pinch of salt and pepper

Optional: lettuce as a nice base, but not necessary

METHOD

Throw into a bowl almost anything that can be cut into bite-size pieces (veggies, protein, herbs), drizzle with olive oil, vinegar, and lemon, and toss all together! Give it a taste to see if it needs anything else. Enjoy!

TASTE TIPS

I have used green beans as my leftover veggie. A half can of black beans lasted for 3 salads. This salad is also great with other canned beans or tuna. Fresh vegetables make it crunchy and delicious.

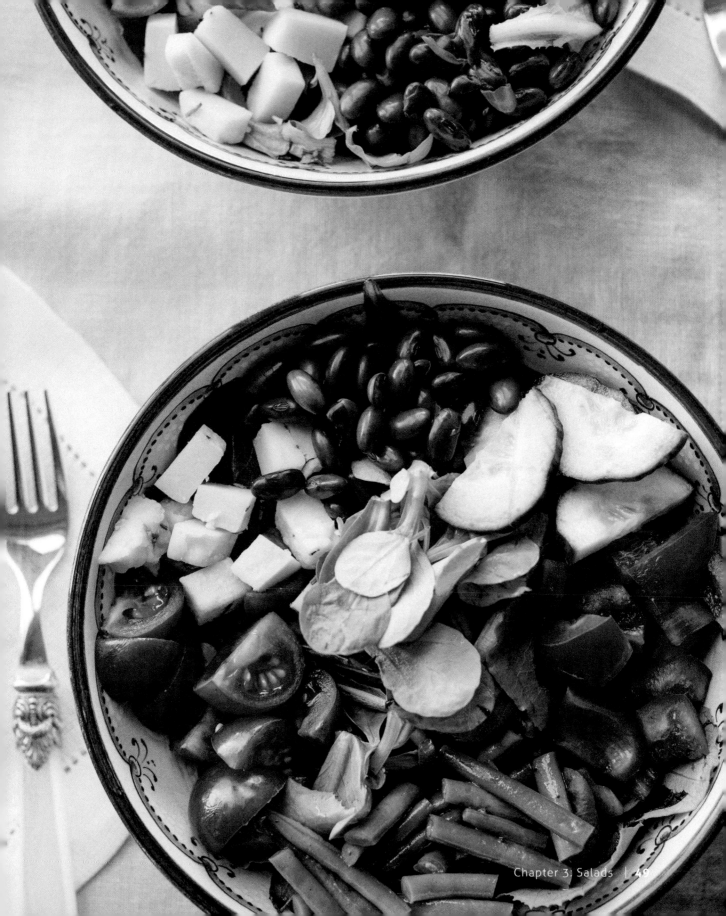

warm street corn salad

This corn was inspired by that yummy street corn-on-the-cob that you find at fairs and in some Mexican and Cuban restaurants. As much as I enjoy this dish, I would rather not have juicy corn and cayenne pepper smeared all over my chin. So, this is a very similar and tasty, if less messy, alternative—off the cob.

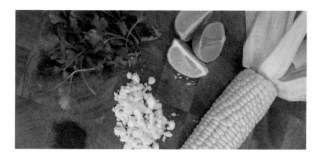

INGREDIENTS

Drizzle of olive oil (for cooking)

A few ears of corn (on the cobs)

A few tablespoons mayonnaise

A few limes (zest and juice)

Handful of crumbled feta or Cotija cheese

Small handful of chopped cilantro leaves

Dash of paprika or cayenne pepper

Dash of salt

METHOD

Drizzle some olive oil in a hot pan. Place the corn (still on the cob) in the pan and brown it on all sides by turning it occasionally while cooking. (Sometimes this takes a while so be patient, it also tends to POP.) When the corn has browned on all sides, remove it from the pan and cut the kernels off the cob, throwing them into a bowl.

In a separate bowl, make the dressing with a few small spoonfuls of a good quality mayonnaise and the juice and zest of a few limes. Pour the dressing over the corn little-by-little to lightly coat it. Add a handful of crumbled feta or Cotija cheese, chopped cilantro, and a dash of paprika or cayenne pepper and salt. Mix everything together and give it a taste!

Herby Egg Salad

MAKES: 2 SERVINGS

Just what it sounds like: egg salad and herbs. WAY better than traditional egg salad. Make it your own.

INGREDIENTS

4 eggs, hard-boiled

2 large spoonfuls of mayonnaise

1 small spoonful of mustard

Very small handful of cilantro leaves (no stems)

4 sprigs of chives

Very small handful of parsley leaves (no stems)

Pinch of salt and pepper

METHOD

Set the eggs in the bottom of a saucepan and put enough water in the pan to just cover the top of the eggs. Place them on high heat until the water starts to boil. (You will hear the eggs rumbling around.) Let the water boil for a minute, then turn off the heat and let the eggs sit in the water for about 10-12 minutes.

Carefully drain out the hot water, and set the eggs in a bowl of cold water.

When the eggs are cool enough to handle, gently tap each one on the side of the counter and peel the shells.

Using a fork or knife, mash the eggs in a bowl, and then add the mayo, mustard, chopped herbs, salt, and pepper. Mix the ingredients together, and taste. Serve this delicious Herby Egg Salad on toasted bread, in a wrap or lettuce cups, or simply eat with a spoon!

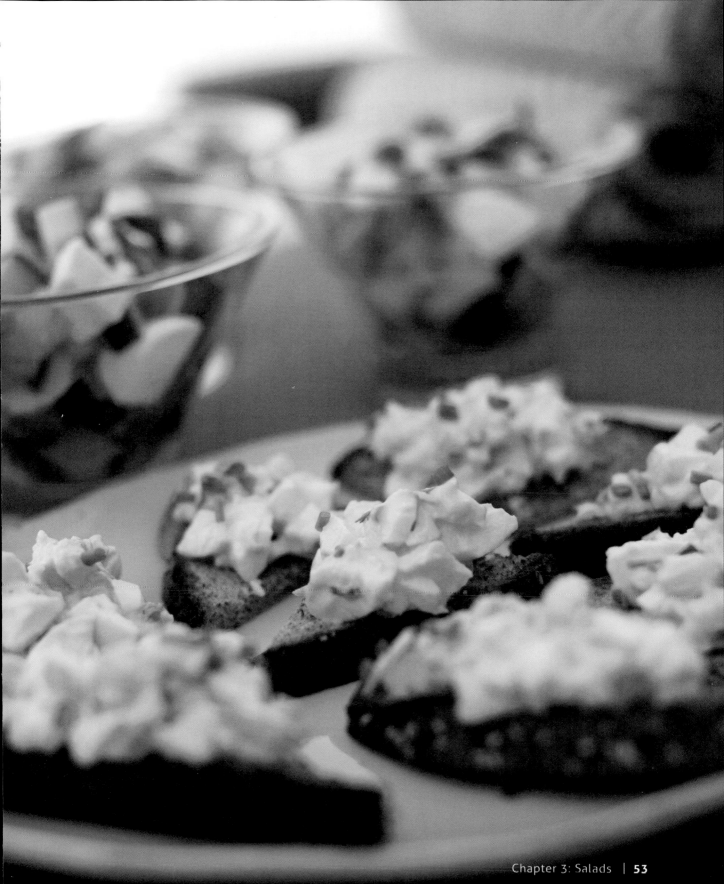

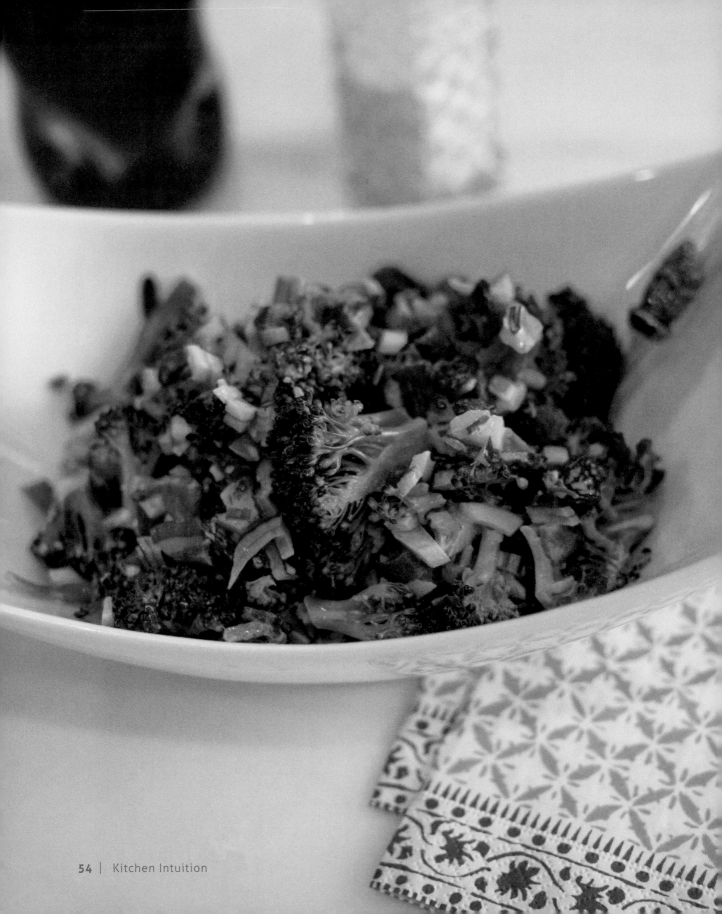

Broccoli SALAD

I know this looks like a strange combination of ingredients, but it is actually an amazing combination of flavors for your taste buds.

INGREDIENTS

A few pieces of bacon

1 tablespoon salt

1 head of broccoli
(cut into small florets)

¼ red onion

Handful of raisins

Splash of apple cider vinegar

Large spoonful of mayonnaise

METHOD

Cook the bacon until it is crispy, and then transfer it from the pan to a plate to cool.

Make a large bowl of ice water for blanching the broccoli immediately after cooking. Heat a pot of salted water to boiling, then add the broccoli florets and cook for 2 or 3 minutes until it turns bright green! When the broccoli is cooked to your preference, drain the hot water and transfer the broccoli into the bowl of cold water to stop itfrom cooking and losing its crunch. (This is called *blanching*.) When the vegetables have cooled, drain the cold water.

Chop or tear up the bacon into crumbly pieces. Dice the onion into small pieces—determining how much raw onion you can tolerate eating! Pour a splash of apple cider vinegar into a cup with a heaping spoonful of a healthy brand of mayo, and mix together until it is a consistency and taste you like. Put the broccoli, onion, bacon, and raisins into a large bowl. Drizzle with the dressing, stirring until all the ingredients are well coated. Enjoy!

TASTE TIP

This is another "even-better-the-next-day" recipe (although sometimes I can't wait that long), which is what makes it great for picnics, home-packed lunches, or as a side dish for gatherings. It is also delicious on the spot.

Veggie salad

This can be made with any vegetable, and you can use leftovers or cook fresh vegetables. It is delicious either way.

INGREDIENTS

1 zucchini

1 asparagus

Any leftover vegetables in your fridge

1 cup of lettuce

1 avocado (chopped or sliced)

Dressing:

¼ cup of olive oil

¼ cup of balsamic vinegar (or apple cider vinegar)

1 large spoonful of a good quality mustard

METHOD

I cooked each of the vegetables by first cutting them to the size I like to eat and then grilling them. But you can also pop them into a preheated 375-degree Fahrenheit oven or sauté them on the stove. After cooking, add the vegetables to a bowl with your preferred lettuce and an avocado, and then toss them with this dressing (one of my favorites).

DRESSING

Whisk or blend, then shake in a bottle: olive oil, balsamic vinegar (though apple cider vinegar is great, too), and a big spoonful of a good quality mustard. Drizzle over your Veggie Salad.

TASTE TIP

This salad is also great with corn, squash, sweet potatoes, green beans, broccoli, and literally any vegetable you most enjoy.

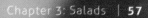

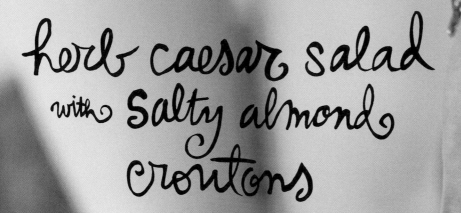

herb caesar salad with salty almond croutons

I don't know why, but I don't like croutons. Yes, I am one of those that don't often eat "gluten" but my dislike for croutons is more than that. I prefer my bread soft and warm rather than stale and crunchy. So I decided to try almonds to add that "crunch factor" to this Caesar salad.

INGREDIENTS

Romaine lettuce (or another crunchy lettuce)

Croutons:

Handful of almonds

1 egg

Pinch of garlic powder

Pinch of salt

Pat of butter, for greasing baking sheet

Dressing:

1 big spoonful of mayonnaise

Drizzle of apple cider vinegar

Drizzle of olive oil

Herbs: basil, cilantro, parsley and tarragon (if fresh, use a small handful of each; if dried, use only a dash of each)

Optional: *pinch of salt and a drop of honey or agave syrup*

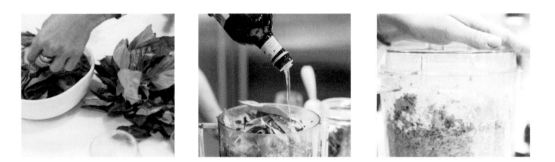

METHOD

Preheat the oven to 350 degrees Fahrenheit.

Place a handful of almonds in the blender or Cuisinart and pulse them until they are crumbly, but *not* too fine. In a bowl, mix together the egg, garlic powder, and salt. On a greased baking sheet, flatten the almond mixture into a layer about a quarter of an inch thick. Place in the oven for a few minutes until golden brown. Meanwhile, wash and chop or tear the lettuce to your liking.

DRESSING

In a blender, mix together the mayo, apple cider vinegar, olive oil, and herbs. (Add less vinegar if you like your dressing thick, and more if you prefer it thinner.) It should be a light green color by the time all the herbs have blended together. Give it a taste. Sometimes at this point I add a pinch of salt or a drop of honey or agave syrup to change up the flavor, depending on my mood.

Add the dressing to the salad and toss all the ingredients together. Once the almond croutons have cooled and hardened, break them up into crumbly bits and add them to the salad.

TOMATO CUCUMBER *Mozzarella* SALAD

INGREDIENTS

Salad:

1 tomato, chopped or a handful of cherry tomatoes

1 ½ cucumbers, chopped into bite-size pieces

1 ball of mozzarella or burrata, cut into bite-size pieces

Handful of basil, chopped

Dressing:

Drizzle of olive oil

Pinch of salt

Optional: *splash of balsamic vinegar, lemon juice*

METHOD

Toss all together and dress.

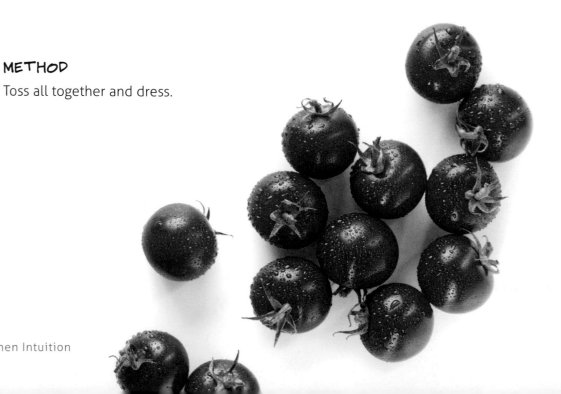

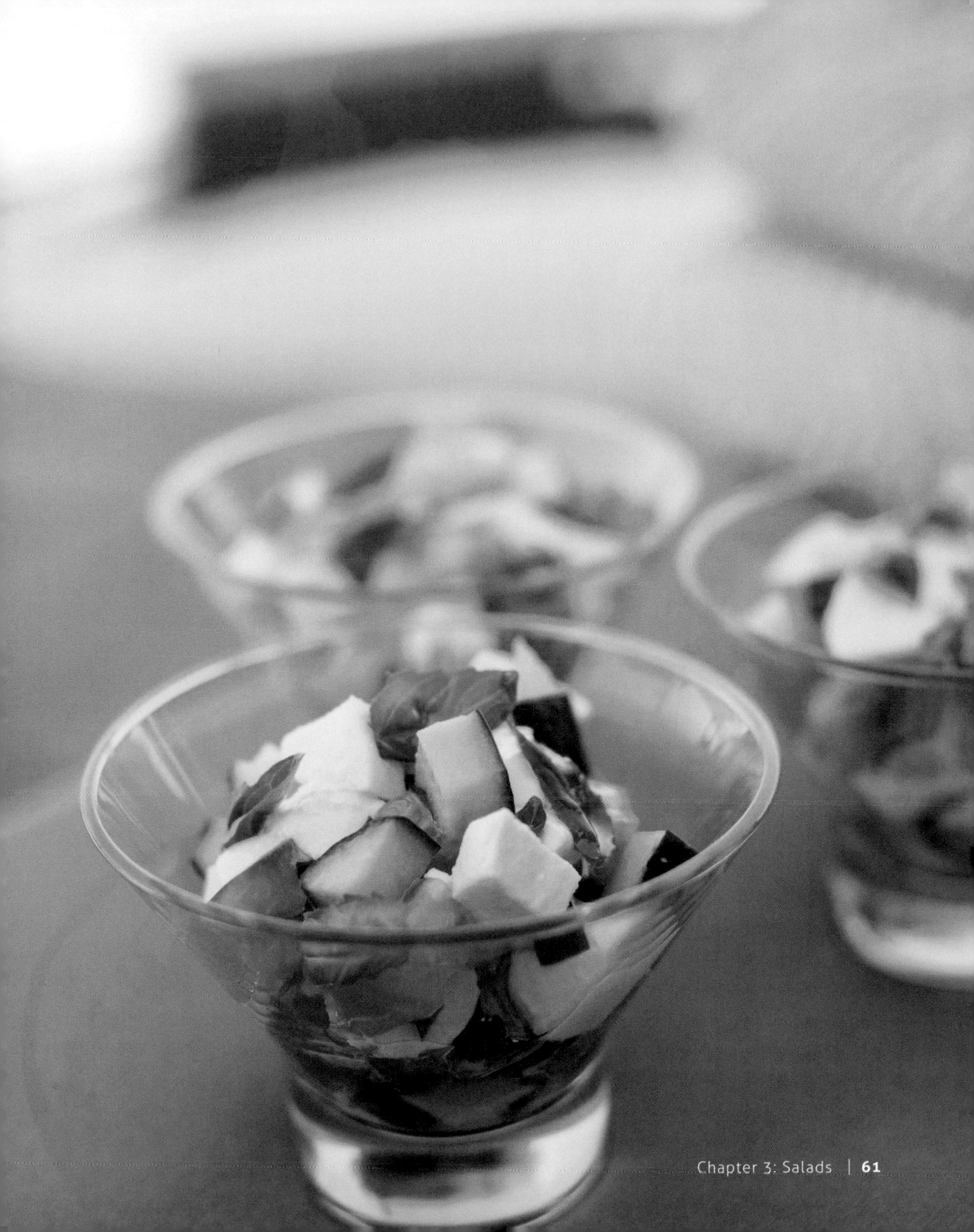

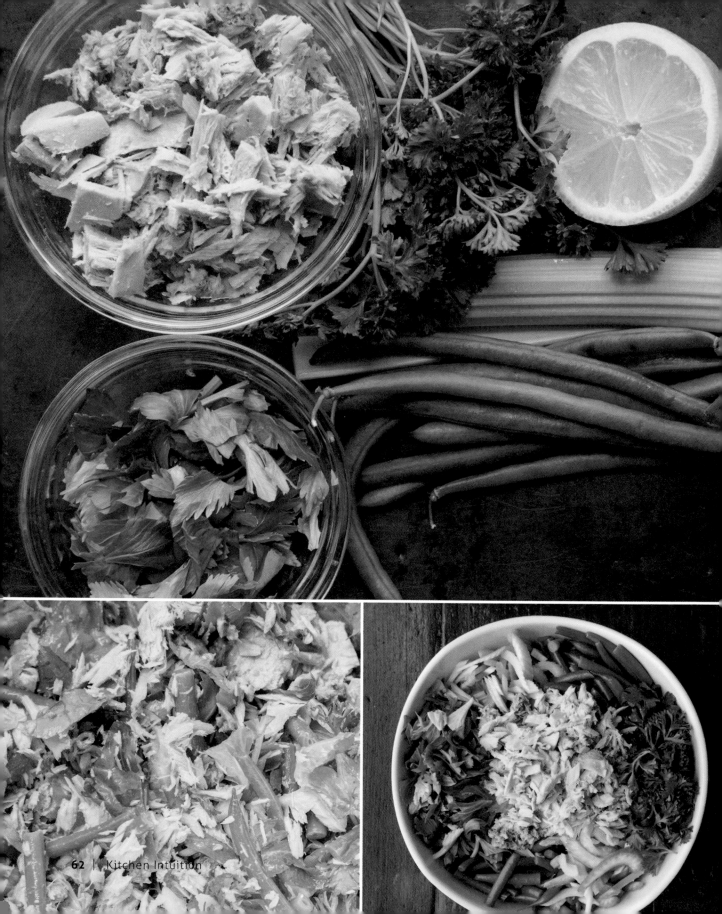

TUNA SALAD
(FIRST DATE SALAD)
SERVES: 2 PEOPLE

I shared this salad, and about half the menu, on a first date. It was one of the best salads I've eaten in a restaurant (and also the best first date I've ever had).

INGREDIENTS

Handful of green beans

Couple pinches of salt

Handful chopped parsley leaves (no stems)

Handful chopped cilantro leaves (no stems)

1 to 2 celery stalks (stalk and leaves—the more leaves the better!)

1 jar or can of tuna

Drizzle of olive oil

2 lemons, juiced

Optional: *2 spoonfuls of capers (highly recommend – although it wasn't on my first date salad)*

METHOD

Boil some water in a saucepan (enough to cover the green beans). While waiting for the water to boil, cut the ends off the green beans and cut them into thirds. When the water boils, add a couple pinches of salt and the green beans. You only need to cook the beans for about 2 minutes. They should still be green and crunchy, but not raw.

Put aside a bowl of cold water with ice cubes for blanching the green beans after they've been cooked and drained from the boiling water.

When the beans are done cooking, use a slotted spoon or strainer to remove the beans from the boiling water, and quickly place them into the ice water. (This is called *blanching* and it works with pretty much any vegetable to stop them from cooking longer after you remove them from the stove. It helps them retain their bright green color and crunchy texture.)

While the beans cool down in the ice water, chop up a few handfuls of parsley and cilantro leaves. (Try other herbs, too, if you like!) Next tear off all the leaves from a bunch of celery (the leaves are what *makes* this tuna salad, so try to get all of them). Then slice the celery on a diagonal as thinly as possible.

Put all the ingredients into a big bowl, including the tuna. (Throw in capers if you like them.) Drizzle the salad with olive oil and the juice of a couple lemons, adding salt to taste. Does this suit your palate? Does it need anything else? Use that intuition!

Fun with Flavor: Working with Herbs and Spices

Spices and herbs are a great way to add flavor, color, and nutritional value to your food. If you find a particular spice, or a combination of spices that you like, try them in some of my recipes. Be bold. Who knows what works until you've tried?

THE DIFFERENCE BETWEEN A SPICE AND AN HERB

Spices are the aromatic parts of plants used for flavoring and coloring food. They are the seed, fruit, bark, berry, bud, or vegetable parts of plants and include the spices cinnamon, nutmeg, garlic, turmeric, cumin, and onion powder, to name a few.

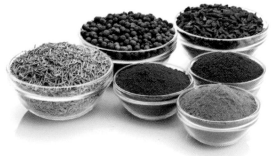

Herbs are the leafy green, often aromatic parts of plants used as medicinals or for seasoning. Examples of herbs include rosemary, thyme, oregano, basil, and parsley.

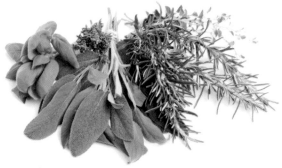

ORIGINS

We've come to identify certain regional food with particular flavors and seasonings. Curry, cumin, and turmeric underlie many Indian recipes. Oregano, basil, and thyme inform many Italian and Mediterranean dishes. Cardamom, five-spice, and certainly cinnamon flavor fond memories of many favorite Asian dishes.

But human migration and the spice trade spread the use and cultivation of herbs and spices across cultural boundaries. Many of these ingredients, as we studied in elementary school, originated in China and Asia, and thanks to Marco Polo and other explorers along the spice trade routes, then spread into the Roman Empire and beyond. There were no hard and fast rules about how to use these new, fragrant spices and herbs—people experimented and incorporated them into their own regional dishes. Many touted some ingredients' medicinal benefits. Ginger originated in China and was used to counter gastrointestinal concerns and motion sickness. Horseradish was used in ancient Greece to treat food poisoning, among other things, and as a cough expectorant in Europe in the middle ages. Many of these natural herbal remedies are still used today.

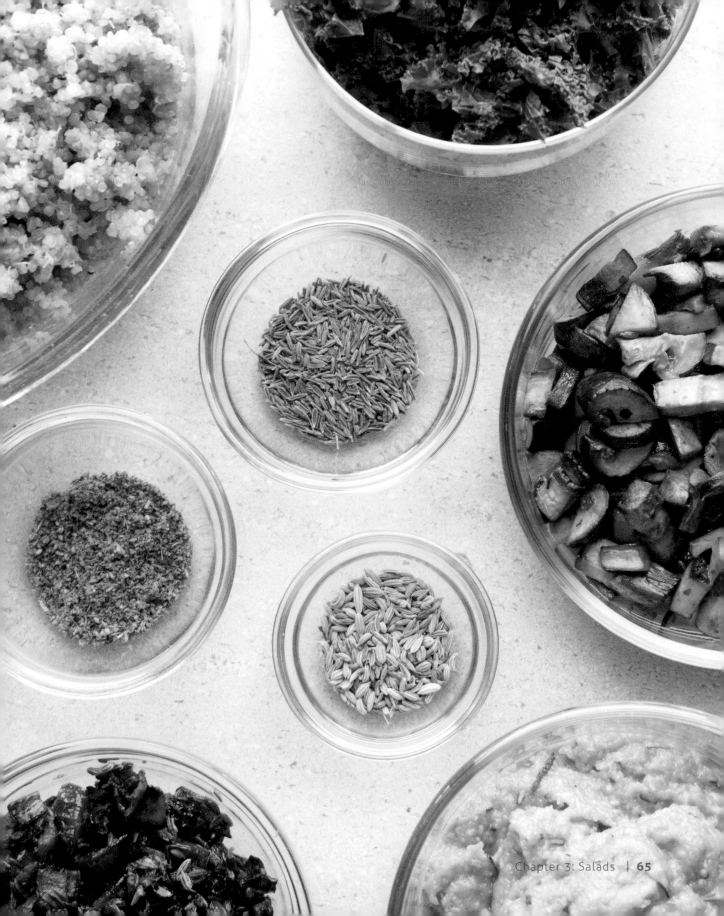

It is fun to learn about the particular seasonings that flavor some of our favorite cultural cuisines, and you will find plenty of opportunities to play with some of these flavors in the recipes in *Kitchen Intuition*. But I also invite you to experiment with spices and herbs that suit your own tastes and to make these recipes your own.

PANTRY PARTY

Invest in a spice collection. You certainly don't need every spice in the world. Start with the ones you most like and expand your collection over time. Bear in mind that spices have a shelf life of only about six months (for freshness), so only buy enough to last that long.

When possible, fresh herbs are also a good investment. You will notice a difference when you begin cooking with fresh (preferably organic) herbs and spices. You may even eliminate unhealthy, processed, and packaged (not to mention expensive) condiments and sauces by substituting spices and herbs instead.

DEVYN'S HERB AND SPICE RACK

The following list of herbs and spices are ones I use regularly when experimenting in my own kitchen. Learning how different cuisines combine different spices and herbs and which ones work best in their particular dishes gives me a great starting point to jump off and explore.

Dried (or fresh) Herbs

Rosemary – Mediterranean shrub in mint family; the narrow gray-green leaves are great for grilling or roasting meat and also in soups and casseroles

Thyme – Eurasian herb or low shrub, also in mint family; leaves used as seasoning (though not much is needed); goes well with lamb, chicken, and pork

Oregano – Eurasian herb, also in mint family; leaves used as seasoning in tomato sauces, Mediterranean, Italian, and Greek dishes

Basil – native to Asia and Africa, also in mint family; leaves used as seasoning, but should be added to sauces near the end of cooking to preserve their flavor

Parsley – Eurasian herb; leaves used as seasoning or garnish; try in soups, sauces, and salads

Cilantro – the fresh stems and leaves of the coriander plant; a nice balance to the spicy ingredients in Mexican dishes

Dill – native to Eurasia; leaves and seeds are often used as seasoning in seafood dishes, salads, and dips

Spices

Many of the following spices can be traced back to their Asian origins, but they can also be found in many other cultural dishes as well.

 Turmeric – strong, bitter flavor, used for color in mustards and curries, but can be added to many dishes

 Nutmeg – nutty, sweet flavor often used to make desserts like pies, puddings, cakes, and cookies

 Cinnamon – described as a sweet-spicy taste, it partners with chocolate and apples and works well in some vegetable and fruit dishes

 Allspice – tastes like a mixture of cloves, cinnamon, and nutmeg; good in savory dishes and with beef and lamb

 Garlic powder – less strong than fresh garlic, with sweeter undertones

 Onion powder – good substitute for onions in some soups and dips; 1 teaspoon is about the same as a small onion

 Cumin – slightly earthy, nutty flavor; used in curries and in taco seasoning

 Cayenne – the spiciest of chili pepper powders (after paprika and chili powder)

 Paprika – a milder, sweeter, and often smoky version of the chili pepper powders

 Curry – a mix of spices generally including cumin, coriander, turmeric (for the yellow color), pepper, mustard, ginger, clove, cardamom, bay leaf, and fenugreek; the spiciness of the curry depends on the level of hot pepper used in the powder

 Pine nuts – the seed of the Mediterranean stone pine; used in Spanish and Italian dishes, such as pesto

Sources: *The American Heritage Dictionary, 5th edition*, Reference.com

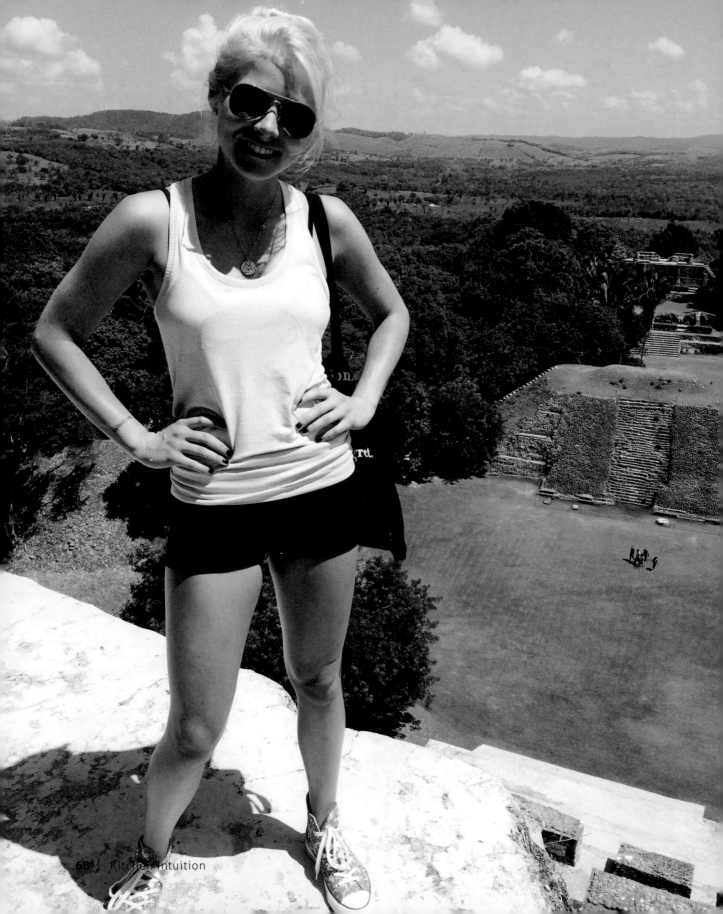

THE DISTINCTIVE FLAVORS OF DIFFERENT CULTURES

The spice trade forever opened borders and minds to new cuisines and cultures, yet even today there are distinctive flavors that underlie many regional dishes. These are just a few, but certainly not all the flavors you might recognize in some of your favorite dishes from abroad.

Mexican – chili (many varieties), chipotle, Mexican oregano, cumin, cilantro, coriander, and clove

Italian – oregano, parsley, garlic, pepper flakes, basil, thyme

Greek – dill, parsley, saffron, lemon, thyme, rosemary, sage

Asian – ginger, garlic, cardamom, fenugreek, five-spice, turmeric, cloves

Indian – cumin, turmeric, coriander, curry, garam masala (usually a blend of cinnamon, cardamom, cloves, cumin, coriander, nutmeg, and peppercorns)

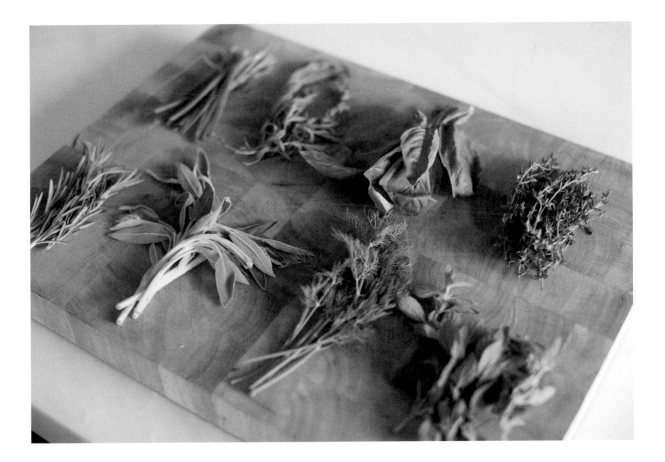

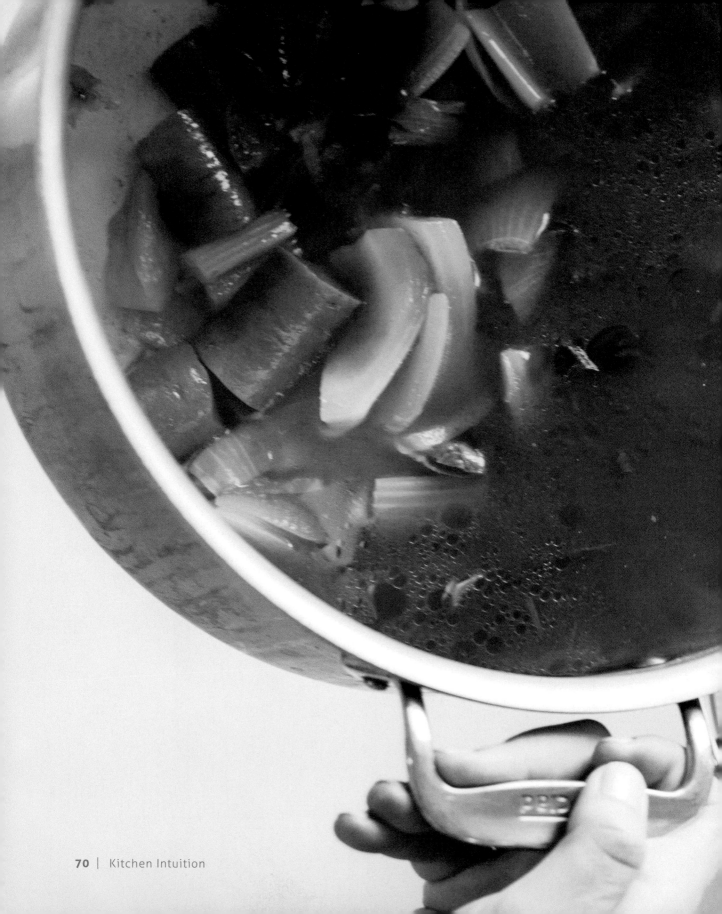

CHAPTER 4

Soups & Bowls

Kitchen Story: Nourishing Body and Soul

Our relationship with food falls somewhere on a spectrum between physical need, a healthy awareness, and psychological obsession. To some degree, we are all aware of the effect food has on our system; whether we are focused on our health, weight, energy, or appearance. You could say that we all follow our own "food religion" with beliefs that are sometimes tied, inexplicably, more to our emotions than scientific fact. Medical conditions like anorexia, bulimia, and orthorexia exist on the extreme end of the psychological spectrum. Thankfully, most of us fall somewhere in the middle of that spectrum with respect to food. However, striking a healthy balance between an appropriate appreciation versus obsession requires mindfulness.

I watched one of my best friends, Lolita, recover from an eating disorder. She was on a difficult journey for a couple years before beginning to understand and accept her body and to see food in a new, healthier way. Living close to one another, I paid close attention to her experience, so that I could learn how to lovingly support her. Although I have no formal training to coach someone through the recovery of an eating disorder, my intuition somehow aligned with her nutritionist's advice. I began simply by eating slowly and mindfully in front of her. My goal, without drawing too much attention to it, was to make food a positive, nourishing experience. In hindsight, I realize that slowing down and doing this "for her" was beneficial for me as well. It was what I needed to continue my own path towards health. I appreciate her for this gift.

Despite her anxiety about having to make too many food choices, I gently urged her to join me in grocery shopping on the nights that I cooked for us. I encouraged her to touch the vegetables as we selected them and would ask if there was anything her body was craving that night. She watched at the counter in my apartment as I grated ginger or minced garlic, sautéed onions and roasted vegetables. I unconsciously slipped in little lessons about what I was cooking as we laughed about college graduation and chatted about our favorite television shows. I wanted her to enjoy the entire experience of food even though she wasn't yet up to cooking for herself.

I hoped she was beginning to notice the difference between making a meal versus pressing a few buttons and ordering food online. It took months of such nights, coupled with the inspiring support of her boyfriend and nutritionist. This turned out to be one of our fondest memories, when we enjoyed the most laughs and the best conversations. Then one morning she sent me a text message with a photograph of a dish she created with the caption, "Look what I made all by myself! The food feels so good in my body!" She had turned a corner. She is an inspiration, and I'm so grateful for her trust and the lesson this taught me—listen to my own instincts when it comes to nourishment and friendship.

Lolita is an example of how I wish to have this book affect others. Simply through encouraging her, asking questions, and leading by example, I unconsciously motivated her to try something new. She bravely got herself into the kitchen. Considering the state she was in, if she could find a way to enjoy a meal that she cooked for herself, ANY of us can.

This experience also showed me how important a role food plays in my relationships. It gave my friend and I a chance to connect each night, to learn from one another and to slow down. Those are the nights we went to bed early, drank only a *few* small glasses of wine, and strengthened our friendship. All thanks to the rituals of connecting through cooking and eating food that nourishes us, body and soul.

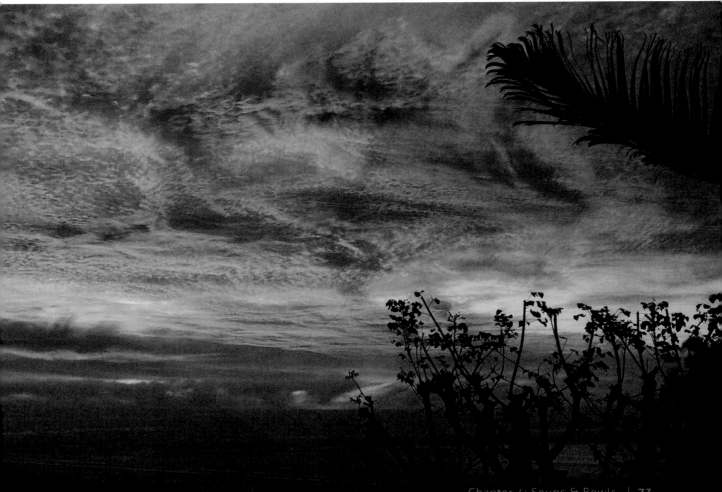

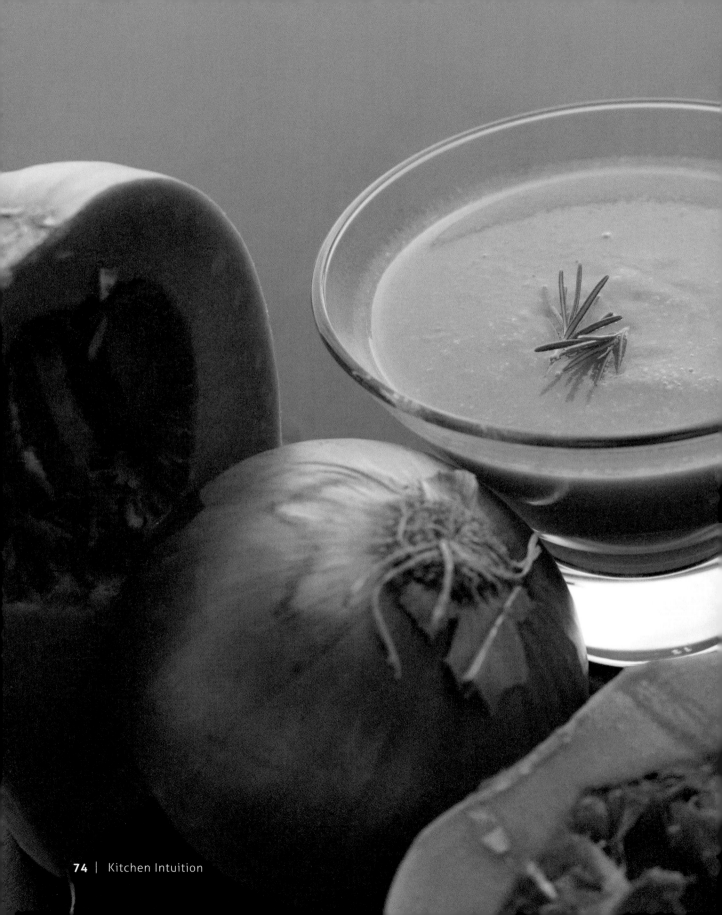

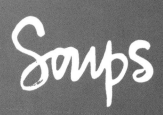

Soups

Easy, warm, and delicious.

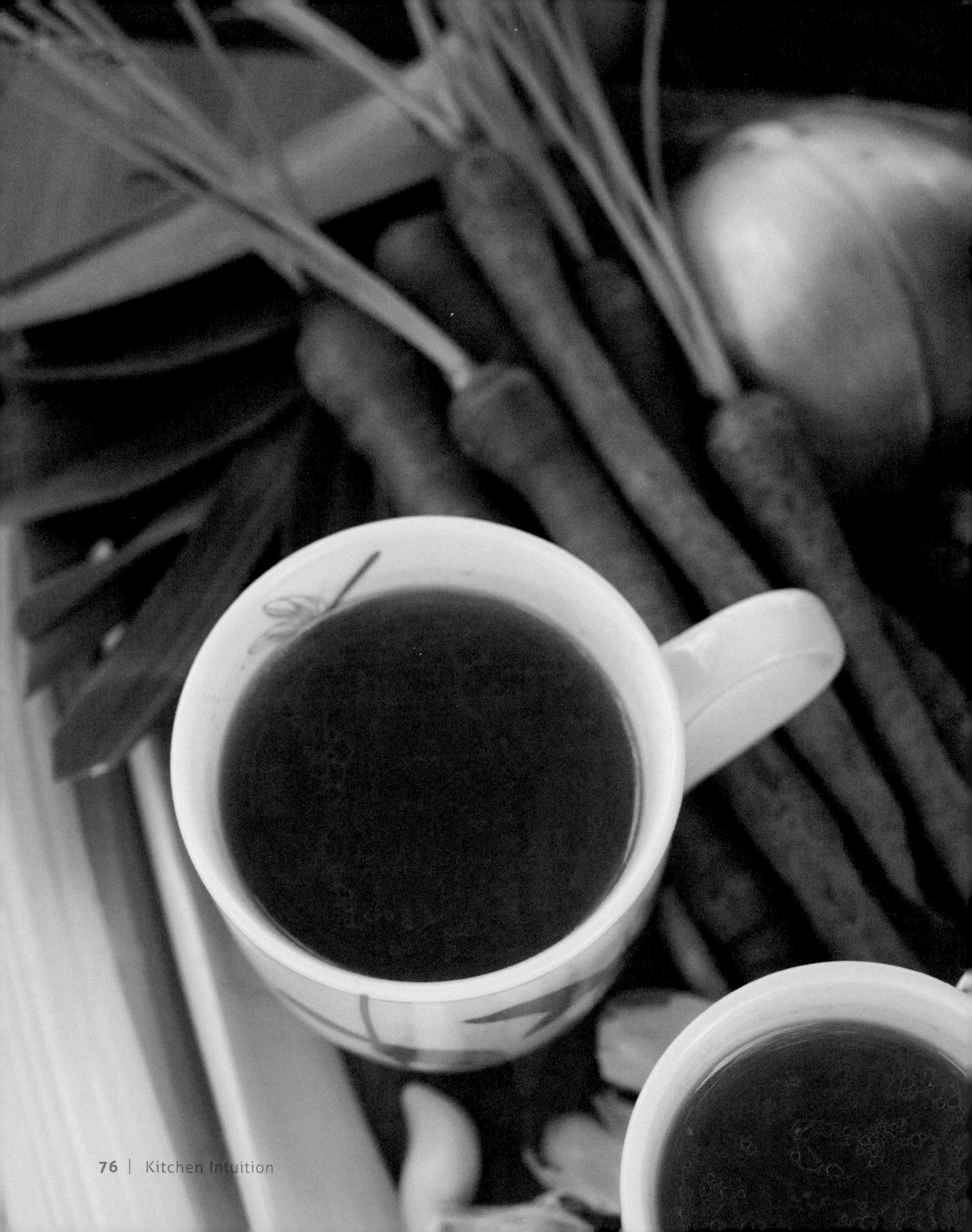

VEGGIE Broth

I would sip on broth all day if it was around. Broth is warm, full of nutrients, tasty, and good to use as a base for other soups, cooking stir-fried veggies, or even in place of water when cooking rice and quinoa.

INGREDIENTS

5 to 10 stalks of celery

1 onion

1 bulb of fennel

3 to 5 carrots

1 leek

Spoonful of coconut oil (or butter, ghee, olive oil, avocado oil)

3 cloves of garlic

Small spoon of turmeric powder

A few sprigs of rosemary (fresh or dried)

Optional: parsley, bay leaves

METHOD

Roughly chop the celery, onion, fennel, and carrots into big chunks. Wash the leek because they can be a little sandy. Cut off the top of the leek and slice only the white and light green part.

In a large pot, throw the veggies in with the coconut oil and stir them around until they start to soften. Add the cloves of garlic and the turmeric powder. Stir for another minute or two.

Now fill three-fourths of the pot with water, add the rosemary, and let it come to a boil. Cover and simmer on low heat for 30 to 60 minutes. Strain the veggie broth by using a slotted spoon to remove the vegetables. Or, you can put a strainer in a large pot in the sink and pour the contents of your veggie soup into the strainer.

Discard or compost the cooked veggies but save the broth that filters through the strainer and collects in the pot below. Salt to taste. When cooled, store in the fridge for future use.

TASTE TIP

Sometimes I add lemongrass, curry powder, red pepper flakes, other vegetables, or even slices of ginger to the mixture when cooking. Check in with your intuition about what your body is craving and try it out!

Bone Broth

INGREDIENTS

3 pounds of grass-fed beef bones

2 carrots

3 celery stalks

2 onions

1 fennel bulb

A few sprigs of rosemary

A few cups of water

Pinch of salt

Drizzle of coconut oil

METHOD

Preheat the oven to 375 to 400 degrees Fahrenheit. Place the bones on a roasting tray, drizzle with coconut oil, and roast them for 30 to 40 minutes, checking halfway through for doneness.

While the bones are roasting, chop the carrots, celery stalks, onions, and fennel bulb into large chunks. Add them to a crockpot with the bones, rosemary, and a few pinches of salt and cover with a few cups of water (enough to cover all the ingredients). Cook the broth for 12 to 24 hours on low. When the broth is ready, cool and strain. Drink immediately or freeze for later use. This broth is great for soups, vegetables, or just plain sipping.

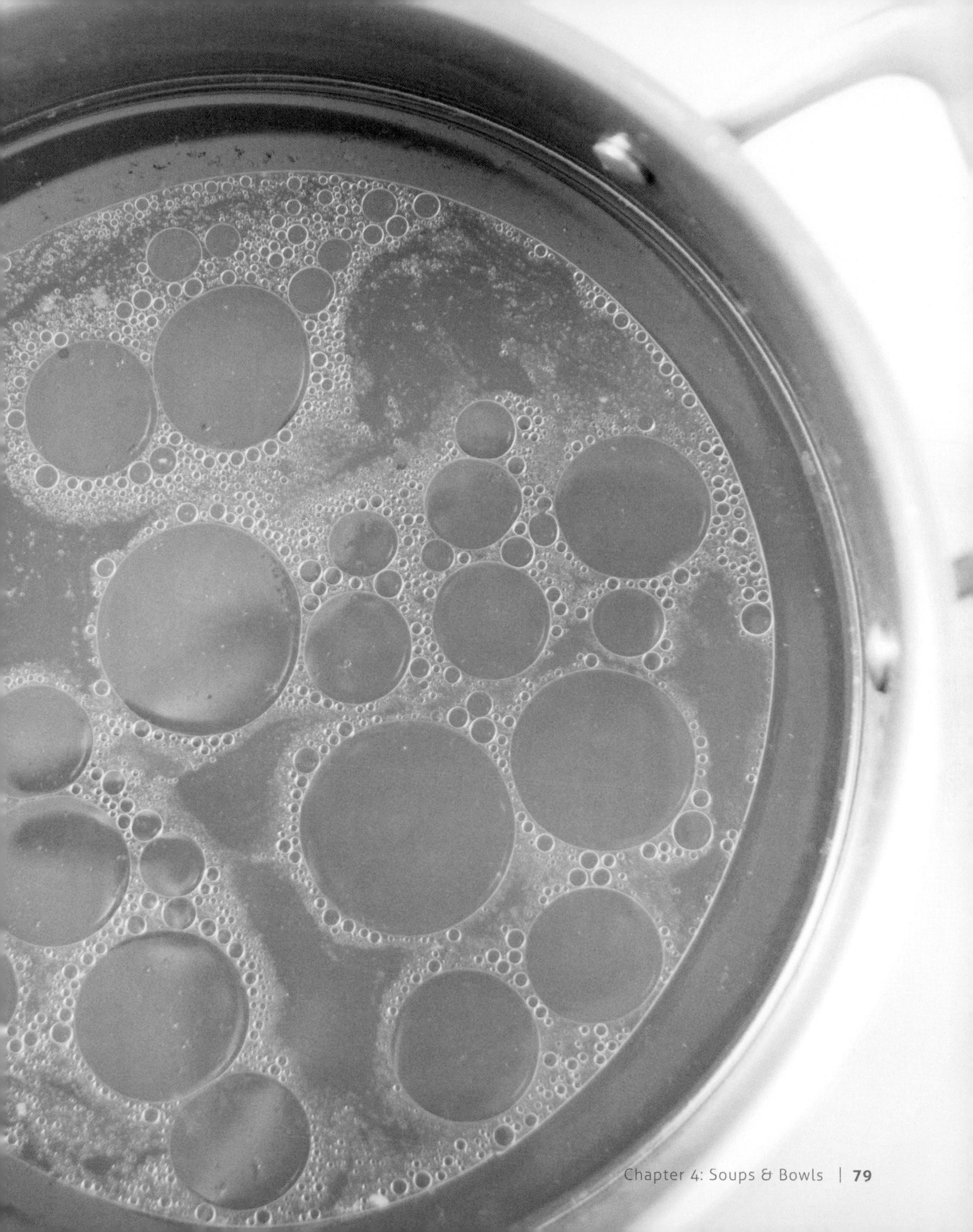

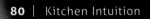

Mushroom SOUP

INGREDIENTS

Lots of mushrooms (Try shitake, portabella, button, baby bella, oyster, maitaki, or a combination of them!)

2 onions

2 tablespoons butter

Thyme (fresh or dried)

Nut milk (or regular milk)

3 cups of broth

Pinch of salt and pepper

Optional: 2 spoonfuls of cream

METHOD

Chop the onions and sauté them in a large preheated pot with 2 tablespoons of butter until they are translucent. The onions will start to soften, and the softer they are, the better the soup will taste; but try not to let them burn.

While the onions are cooking, slice the mushrooms and add them to the pan. You may need to add more butter at this point. You can also add a large pinch of thyme. Continue cooking the mushrooms and onions for about 15 minutes or until both are extremely soft and cooked through. Remove about one-half cup of the mixture from the pot and set it aside. (You will add it back into the soup when it is done.)

Now get out the blender. Put the rest of your onion and mushroom mixture into the blender and slowly add the broth. Blend until smooth. Add broth depending on what mushrooms you used, how many, and how thick you like your soup. (Add more broth for a thinner soup, less broth for thicker.) Pour the blended mixture back into the pot and cook on low heat. At this point I usually add about a half cup of milk (I use almond) and 2 spoonfuls of cream. I add the salt and pepper and return the onions and mushrooms that I set aside earlier. Stir, taste, add... Stir, taste, add... until the soup is your desired flavor and consistency.

TASTE TIP

You don't *have* to set aside the half-cup of sautéed mushrooms and onions in the beginning. I just do that because I like to have a little texture in my soup, something to chew on.

coconut curry butternut squash soup

INGREDIENTS

1 butternut squash

1 cup coconut milk

4 to 5 cups of chicken broth (beef, bone, or vegetable broth is fine, too)

1 white or yellow onion

1 tablespoon butter

1 spoonful curry paste (or powder)

Small spoonful ginger (preferably fresh, grated)

METHOD

Peel the outer skin of the butternut squash and cut it down the middle. Be sure to scrape out the seeds. Chop the squash into cubes. (Sometimes a good potato peeler can help peel the squash.)

Pour the coconut milk and chicken broth into a pot (approximately 1 cup or part of milk to 4 or 5 cups or parts chicken broth). If you are making a small batch of soup, use less milk and chicken broth, but keep the same proportions. Add the peeled, cubed squash to the pot of coconut milk and chicken broth and bring it to a boil. Once it boils, turn the temperature to low and continue cooking until the squash is fork tender.

While the squash is cooking, chop up an onion into pretty small chunks, although the size doesn't matter too much. This is because after it is cooked, you will blend the onion and the squash in a blender or food processor.

Heat up a pan with some butter, add the onion and a pinch of salt, and cook on low for approximately 10 minutes or until the onion is soft and translucent. When the onion is almost done, add a generous amount of curry paste or curry powder to the pan and stir. Peel and grate some ginger (more if you like that spicy, gingery taste—but be careful, it has a rather strong flavor). Add the ginger to the pan with the onions and curry.

When the squash is fork tender and the onions are translucent, take out the blender or food processor. Using a slotted spoon (to strain the liquid from the veggies), remove the cooked squash and transfer it to the blender/food processor. (Save the liquid to blend into the soup as you go. While adding some liquid from the soup into the blender/food processor is fine at this point, it is better to first blend the cooked veggies and then add in broth/liquid as you go.) Blend in the sautéed onions. The mixture in the blender/food processor should be the consistency of mashed potatoes.

Add the broth (leftover from cooking the squash), one cup at a time, depending on how thick you like your soup. It will be hot from cooking, so be careful when blending or tasting. It is a good idea to taste and adjust spices as you go, for instance, you may want to add salt. Trust your intuition.

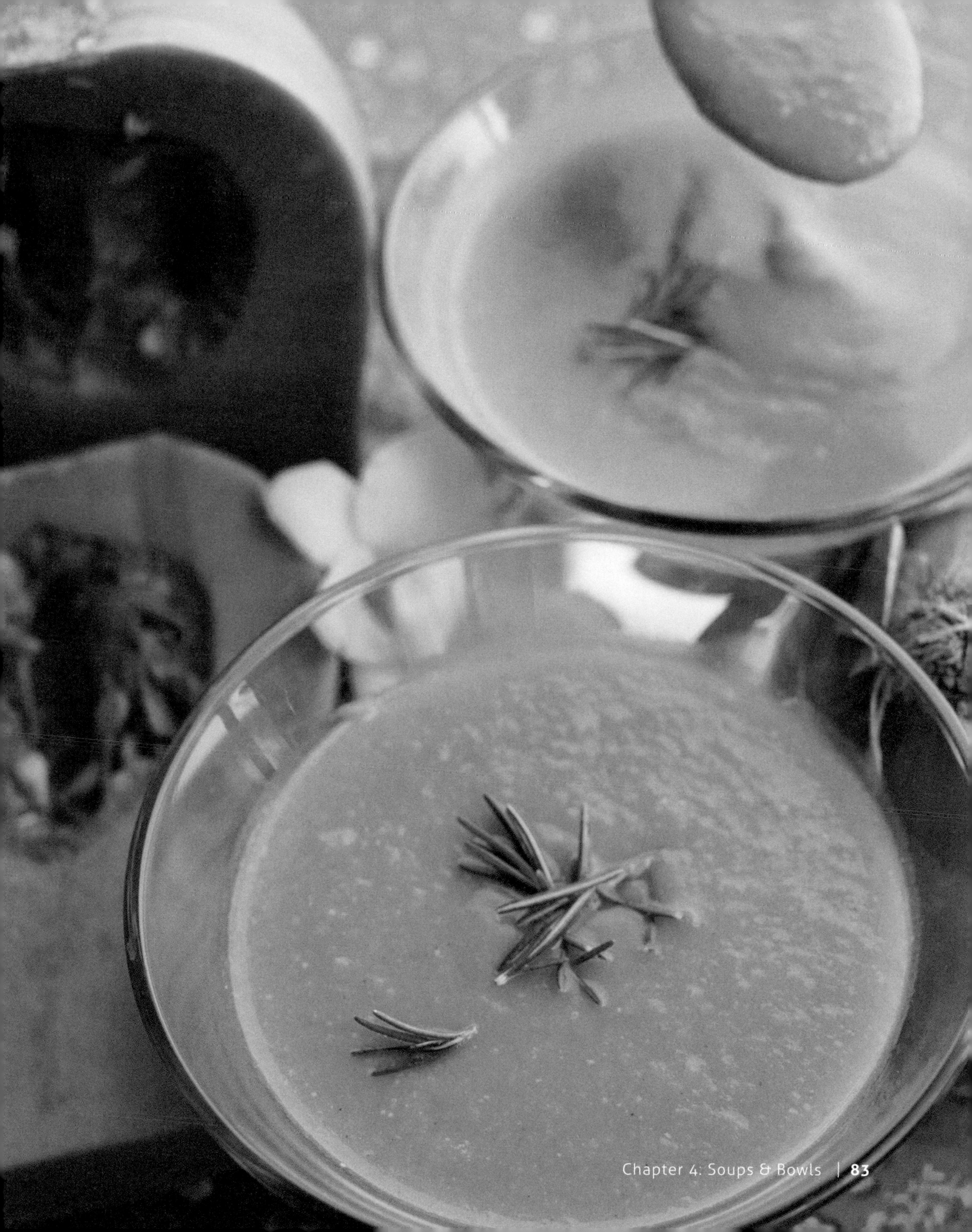

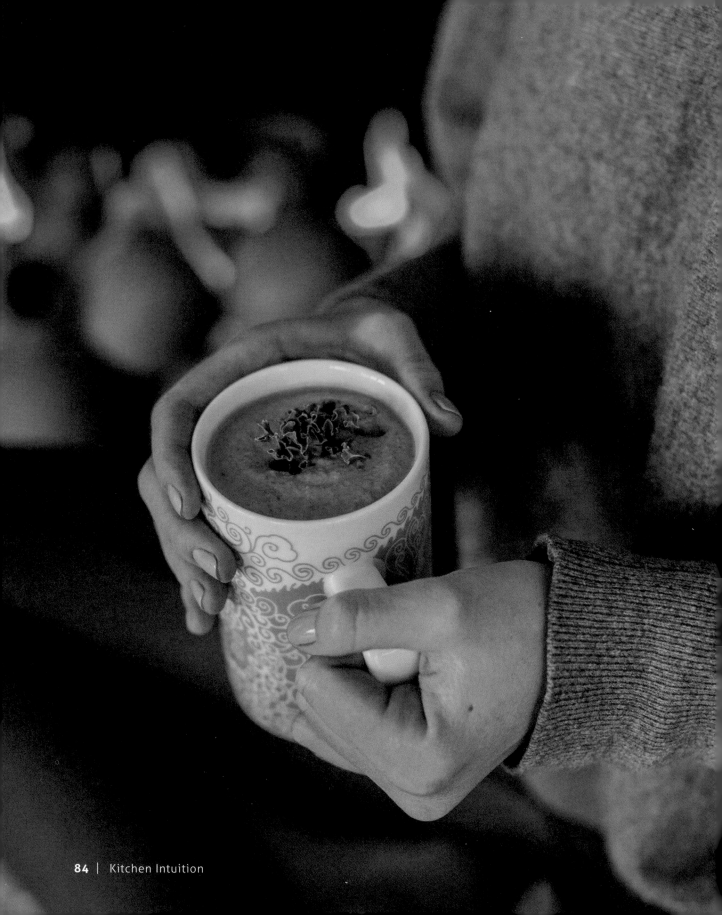

Broccoli Kale Soup

INGREDIENTS

2 bunches of broccoli

2 bunches of kale

Broth (chicken, veggie, bone—veggie
and bone broth recipes are on pages 77–78)

Dash of salt

Couple tablespoons of butter

Spoonful of apple cider vinegar

METHOD

Cut the bottom inch or two off the broccoli, and chop up the rest for cooking. Add the broccoli to a stockpot with enough broth to cover it, and cook to boiling over high heat. Then turn down the heat, and let simmer. Tear off the kale leaves and add them to the warm broth mixture. Keep simmering until the broccoli is fork tender. Carefully transfer the cooked greens to a blender with a slotted spoon. Slowly add in the broth to the blender until the mixture is your ideal soupy texture. Add some salt to taste, about 2 tablespoons of butter, a spoonful of apple cider vinegar, and blend again. Enjoy!

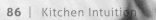

Mushroom Soup

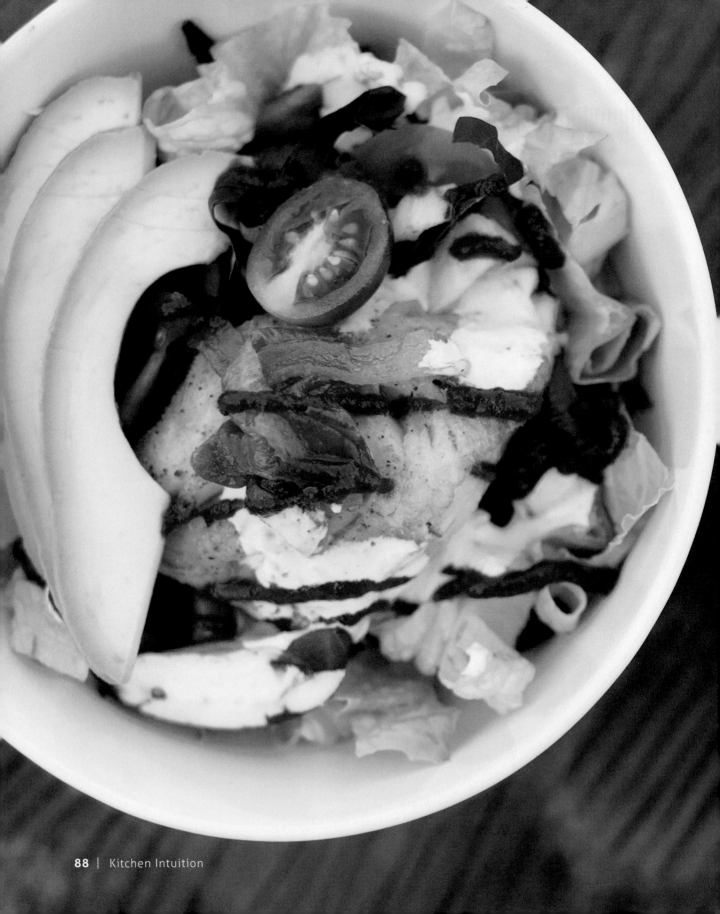

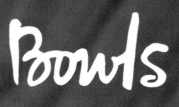

Bowls

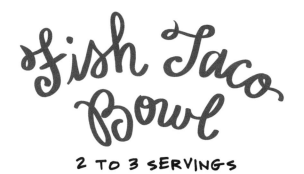

Fish Taco Bowl

2 TO 3 SERVINGS

I love fish tacos but I don't always want to make my own healthy tortillas from scratch. As much as I love eating them in lettuce wraps, they're always falling apart, and I don't feel satisfied. So instead, I just put all the taco goodness into a bowl and eat it up without getting taco sauce running down my sleeve.

INGREDIENTS

For the fish tacos:

½ pound of skinned, boned, and cleaned fish (halibut, mahi-mahi, tilapia, salmon, cod)

1 onion, sliced

Dash of salt

Dash of lemon pepper

Handful of cherry tomatoes

A few leaves of lettuce (romaine, butter, or mixed greens)

Handful of grated cheese

1 avocado

For the taco sauce:

A few cloves of garlic

A few spoonfuls of a healthier mayonnaise

1 lemon or lime, juiced and zest

Dash of salt and pepper

METHOD

Slice the onion into round pieces (like onion rings) and sauté them in a hot, oiled pan with a pinch of salt. Cook them until they start to get soft—but not all the way.

While the onions are cooking, cut your fish into large cubes. (It breaks apart in the pan, so no worries.) Put the fish in the pan with the onions and stir in some spices. (I like salt and lemon pepper. Feel free to experiment.) Keep an eye on the fish; it only takes a few minutes to cook.

While the fish is cooking, slice the cherry tomatoes in half, chop or tear up some lettuce, grate the cheese, and slice up the avocado.

When the fish is done, you can assemble everything in tortillas for tacos or just throw it all in a bowl. Start with the lettuce and add the veggies and fish. Top with avocado slices, and drizzle the taco sauce over the top. Add hot sauce if that's your thing!

TACO SAUCE

Chop up a few cloves of garlic as small as you can get them. Add a few small spoonfuls of mayo, salt, and the juice and zest of a lemon and/or a lime. (I like lots of zest so I usually zest about 3 limes, but I only juice one of them.)

Mix all the ingredients together using a fork or a whisk until it is the consistency of ranch dressing and the taste is to your liking.

Coconut Curry Chicken

INGREDIENTS

1 chicken breast

Several dashes of salt (for seasoning chicken)

½ onion (white or yellow), chopped

2 tablespoons coconut oil (or butter)

1 small piece of fresh ginger, (peeled and grated)

3 to 5 garlic cloves, (cut small)

2 spoonfuls of curry powder (or paste)

1 small spoonful of turmeric powder

1 can coconut milk

1 cup of white rice (cooked according to packet instructions)

Optional: 1 bell pepper, zucchini or vegetable of choice (chopped)

METHOD

Salt both sides of a chicken breast and cook in a pan on medium-high for a few minutes on each side until cooked through. Chop onion, peppers, zucchini, or any other vegetables you would like to add later. Cook a cup of white rice according to the instructions on the package.

In a warm pan with coconut oil, cook the chopped onions until they soften and become translucent. Add the grated ginger and garlic along with the curry and turmeric, stirring for just a few minutes and adding more coconut oil as needed. (The goal is to lightly cook the garlic without burning it, while warming up those spices–you'll start to smell the intensity.)

Next add in the coconut milk. Heat the coconut milk and let it simmer for a little while until it starts to thicken. Pour the curry sauce into a blender, (making sure it is not too hot) and blend until the mixture is smooth. Taste to see if your taste buds would like more salt, curry, ginger, or maybe even something spicier! Use this as your curry base. Stir the chicken or sautéed vegetables of your choosing into the curry sauce, and serve on top of the cooked rice.

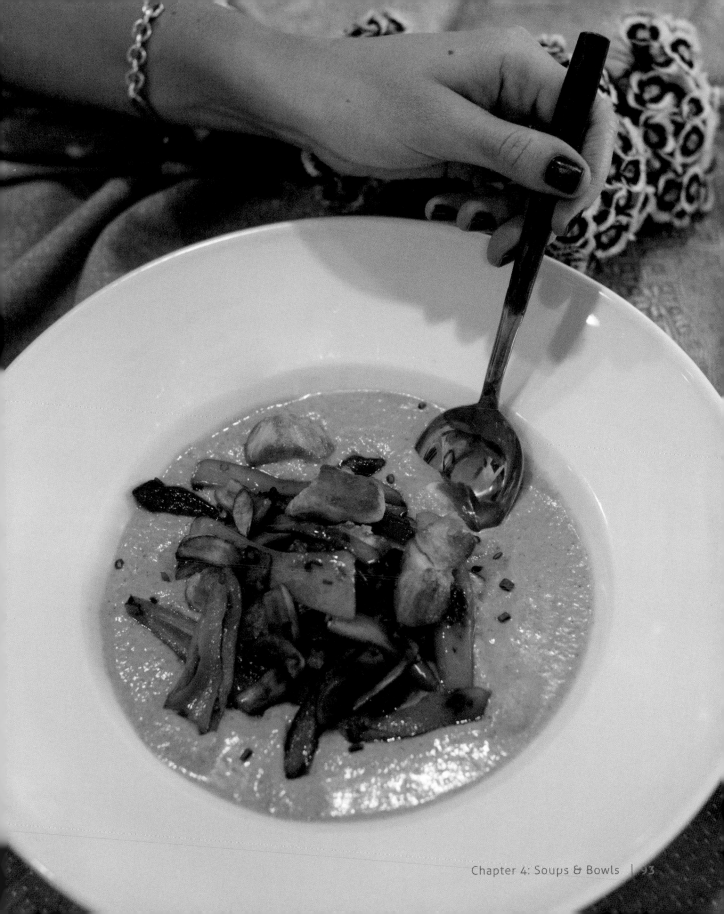

Shrimp Kale Bacon Bowl

INGREDIENTS

Several strips of bacon

Butter (or oil) for sautéing

1 onion, chopped

Several cloves of garlic, chopped

1 bunch kale

4 to 5 shrimp per person

METHOD

Cook the bacon in a pan until crispy, then set it aside to cool.

While the bacon is cooking, chop up the onion and some garlic cloves. In the same pan (with all the bacon fat goodness), sauté the onions and garlic.

Cut or slice out the thick spine of the kale leaves and discard. Then tear up the leaves and add them to the pan with the onions and garlic.

Stir around and cook until the kale and onions are soft. Transfer the cooked kale and onions to a serving bowl.

Use the SAME pan (with all the delicious flavors from the bacon, onion, and garlic) to cook the shrimp. Shrimp should be cooked until they are no longer translucent. This will not take long, so keep an eye on it. (If you bought precooked shrimp, then you are simply reheating them.) Meanwhile, chop or tear up the bacon pieces and sprinkle them into the bowl with the onion, garlic, and kale. Top with the cooked shrimp and enjoy!

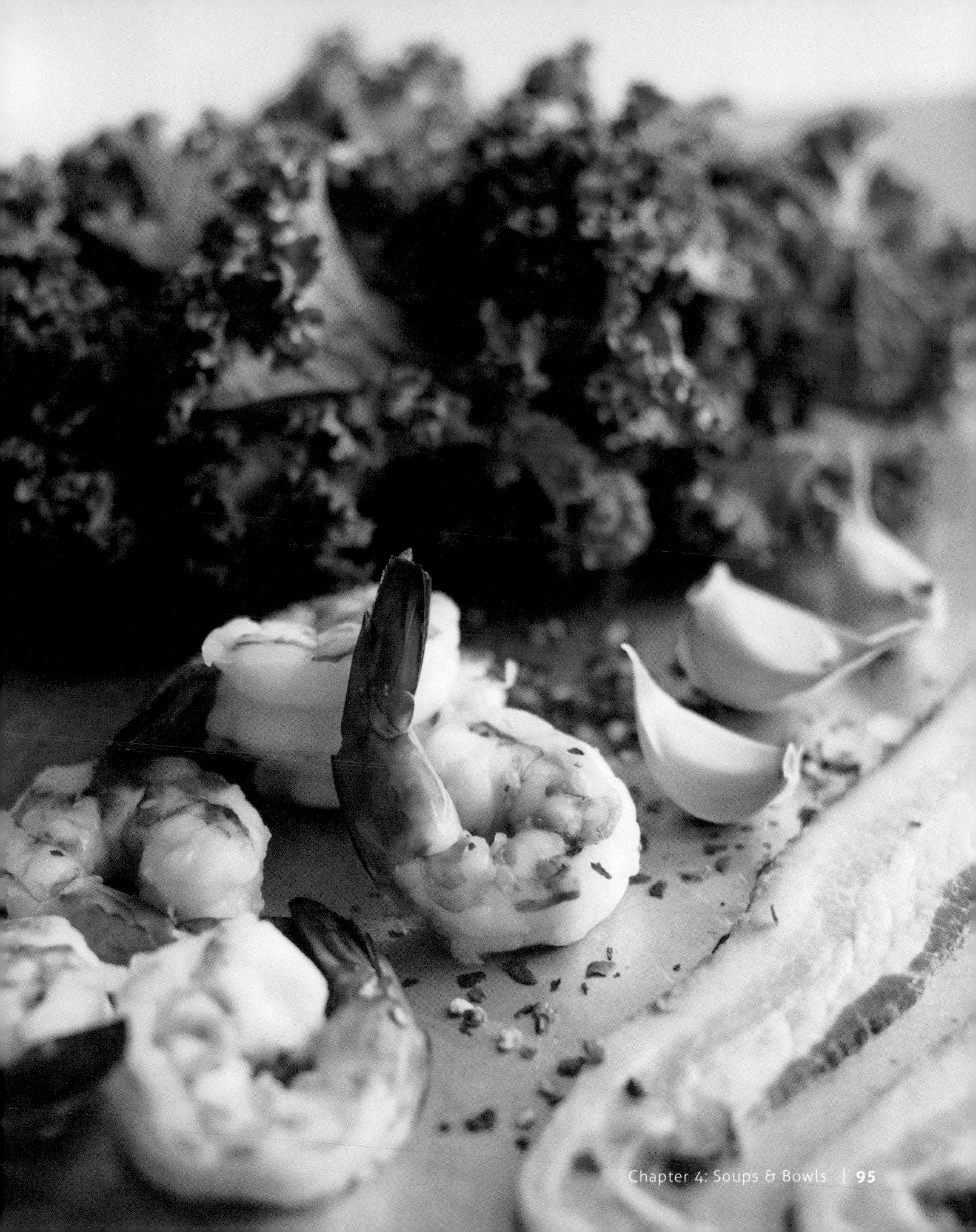

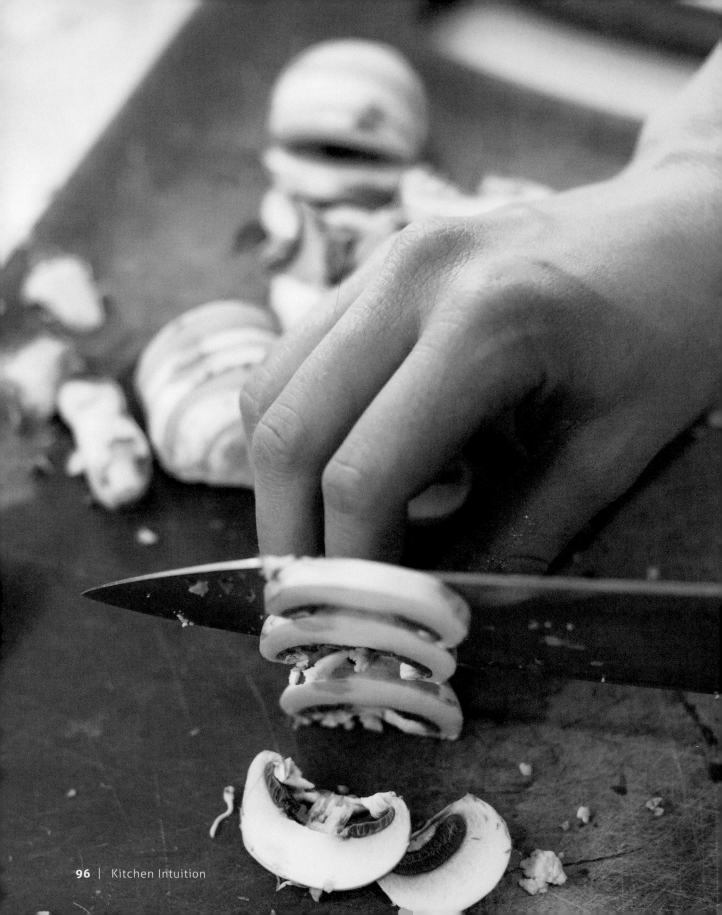

Pizza in a Bowl

*I like this recipe because it has all the delicious flavors of a pizza, but is still something new.
For this recipe, the polenta is made from a boxed cornmeal-like substance, not sliced from the package.*

INGREDIENTS

1 cup polenta

½ cup sun-dried tomatoes

Small handful of mushrooms, sliced

Small handful of mozzarella cheese, grated

Small handful of chopped basil leaves

Handful of fresh, chopped tomatoes

Substitutions
*Use any meat, vegetable or cheese your heart desires.
Make this fun, be creative, and enjoy!*

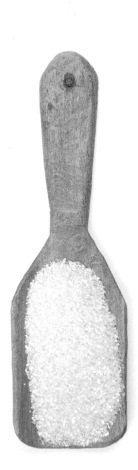

METHOD

Cook about a cup of polenta per person according to the package directions. Assemble in a bowl with a variety of pizza toppings. Think of the polenta as your pizza "crust" substitution. This time I used sun-dried tomatoes, lightly cooked mushrooms, grated mozzarella cheese, basil, and fresh tomatoes.

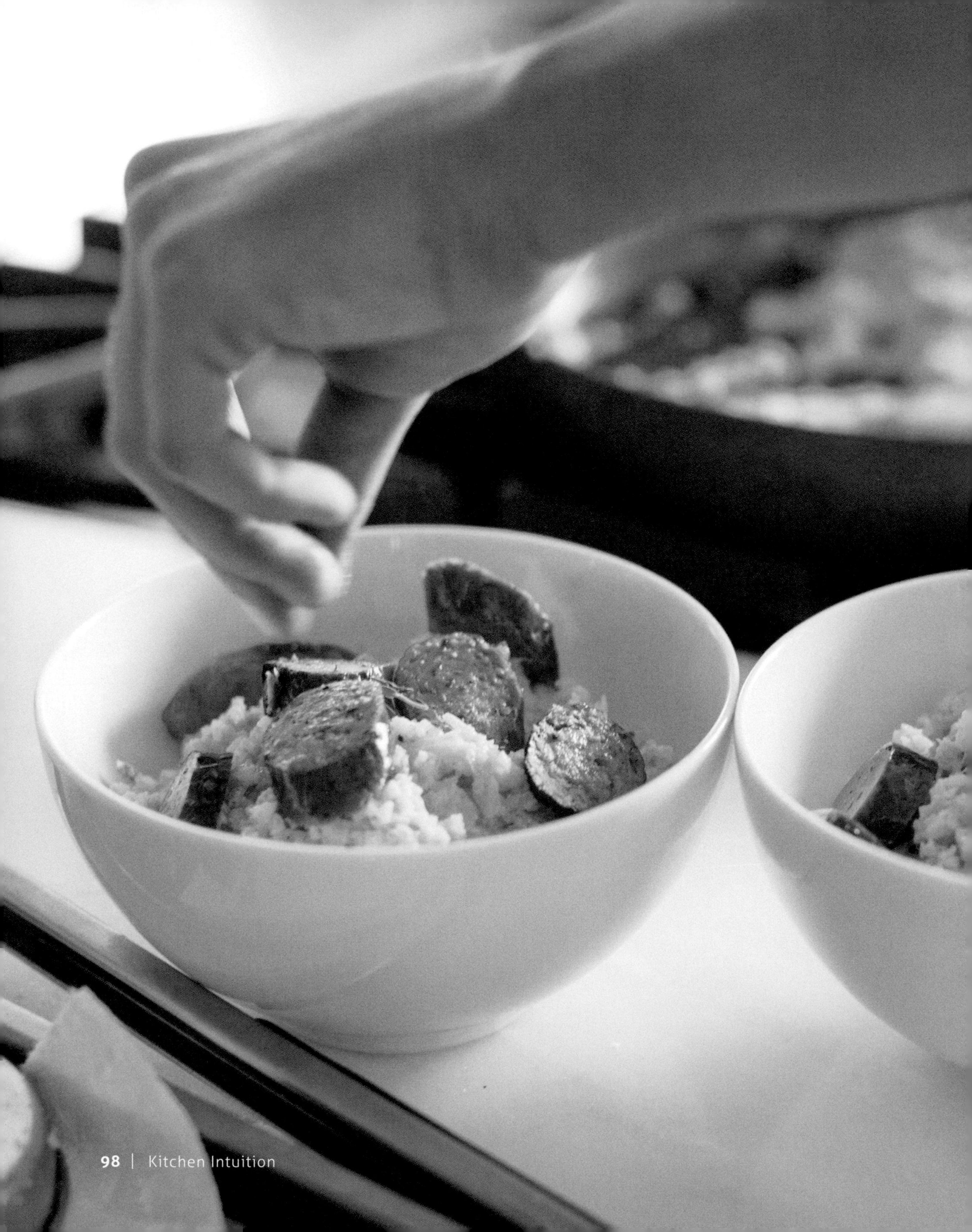

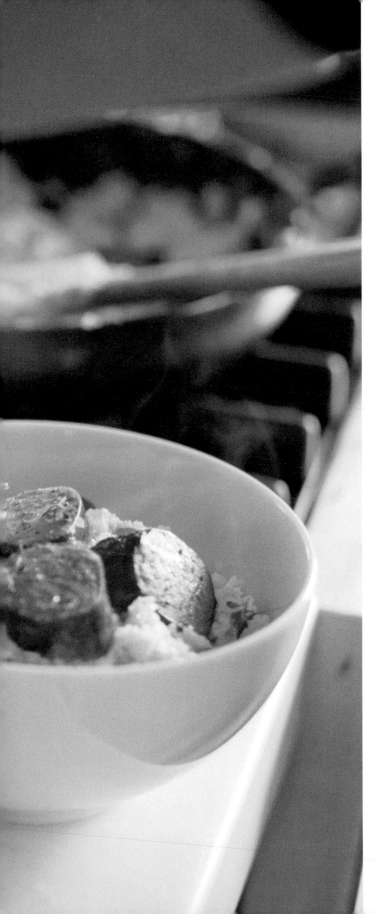

The Cauliflower Risotto Fail

So I thought I had this brilliant idea to try to make a "rice-free" risotto. I love both risotto and cauliflower so... it seemed like a natural. A traditional risotto is more or less made with rice, broth, butter, cream, Parmesan cheese and white wine. I used all of those ingredients, but it DIDN'T turn out. It even smelled bad. This made for a cool picture, and learning experience, but it was one time my intuition led me astray rather than to an immediate success. That's ok. I forgive myself. It hasn't deterred me from trying again; instead it fueled the fire! I am determined to make a delicious cauliflower risotto.

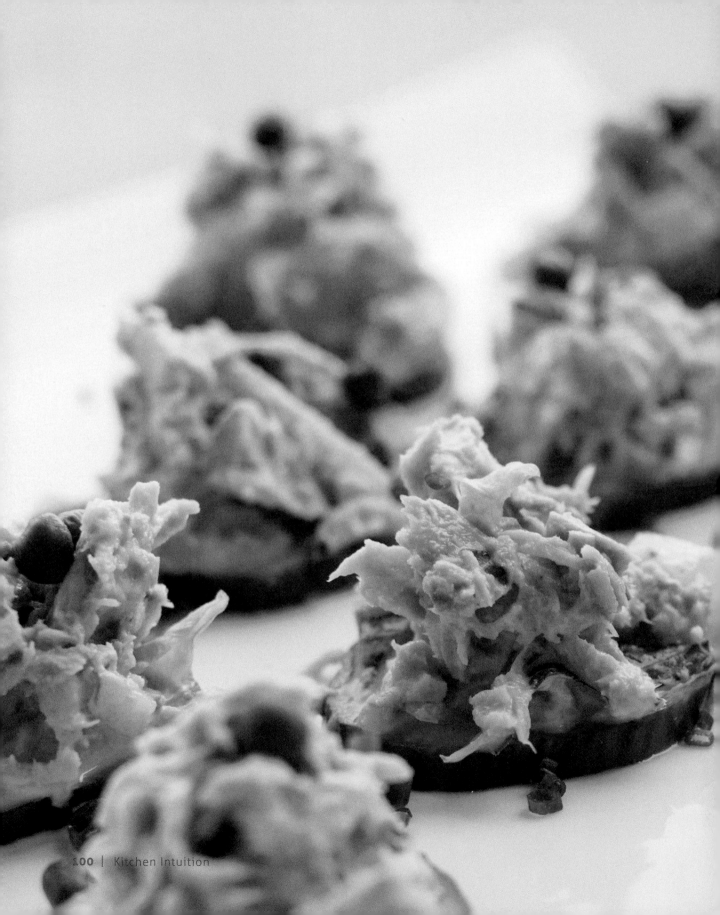

CHAPTER 5

Dips & Bites

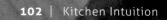

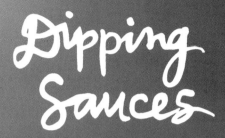

Dipping Sauces

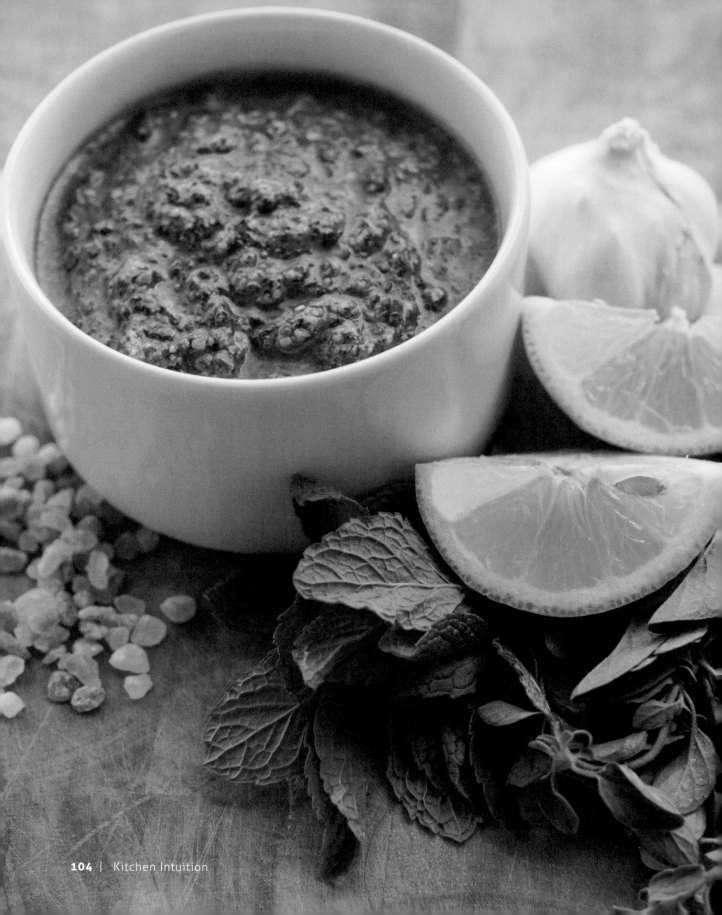

Pesto CHIMICHURRI

This is an Argentinian "pesto" sauce that I put on EVERYTHING. You can dip raw veggies in it or pour it over grilled vegetables, fish, chicken, beef, or even tofu. It adds so much flavor, and the herbs are a healthy alternative to processed sauces.

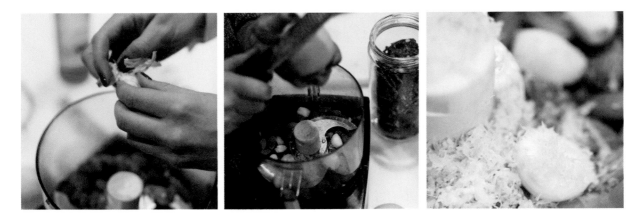

INGREDIENTS

2 to 4 garlic cloves (depending on your love of it)

½ cup olive oil

1 lemon, juiced and zest

1 cup fresh, flat-leaf Italian parsley (no stems)

1 cup fresh cilantro (no stems; can substitute or add in 1 cup basil)

Oregano (small handful if fresh; 1 teaspoon if dried)

¼ to ½ cup red wine vinegar

Dash of salt and pepper

¼ teaspoon chili flakes

Optional: basil

METHOD

In a food processor, blend up a few garlic cloves (depending on how garlicky you like things), with some of the olive oil and lemon zest and juice. Then add in the fresh Italian parsley, cilantro, oregano (if fresh), and a little basil (optional). As you add the fresh herbs into the processor, drizzle in the red wine vinegar and more of the olive oil. Finally, throw in salt, pepper, oregano (if dried), and chili flakes. Keep tasting it as you go until it becomes your desired texture and consistency.

Hummus

This is a huge hit for family parties and sporting events. I also love to use this spread for wraps, sandwiches, and literally anything you can use to dip.

INGREDIENTS

1 can of garbanzo beans

A few dollops of tahini
(sesame seed butter)

A few cloves of garlic

Drizzle of olive oil

Lemon juice

Pinch of salt

METHOD

Drain the garbanzo beans. Add the garbanzo beans, a few dollops of tahini, and a few garlic cloves into a blender or food processor and blend. Add in a few dashes of olive oil (or more if you prefer), some lemon juice (to taste, but not too much at first), and salt, blending until smooth. Depending on how you like your hummus, add more olive oil, tahini, or lemon juice to change the taste and texture. Some people like it thicker for dips and thinner to spread on warps or sandwiches.

TASTE TIP

Like most things, this one took me a few tries to perfect. The taste depends on how sour the lemons, how big the garlic cloves, and what brand of tahini and garbanzo beans I use. I still don't have an exact recipe and it always tastes a little different, but it's still delicious!

Chipotle Lime Hummus

Same as Hummus recipe with the following exceptions:

Substitute lime juice for lemons.

Add canned diced chipotle peppers (only a few; they are spicy)

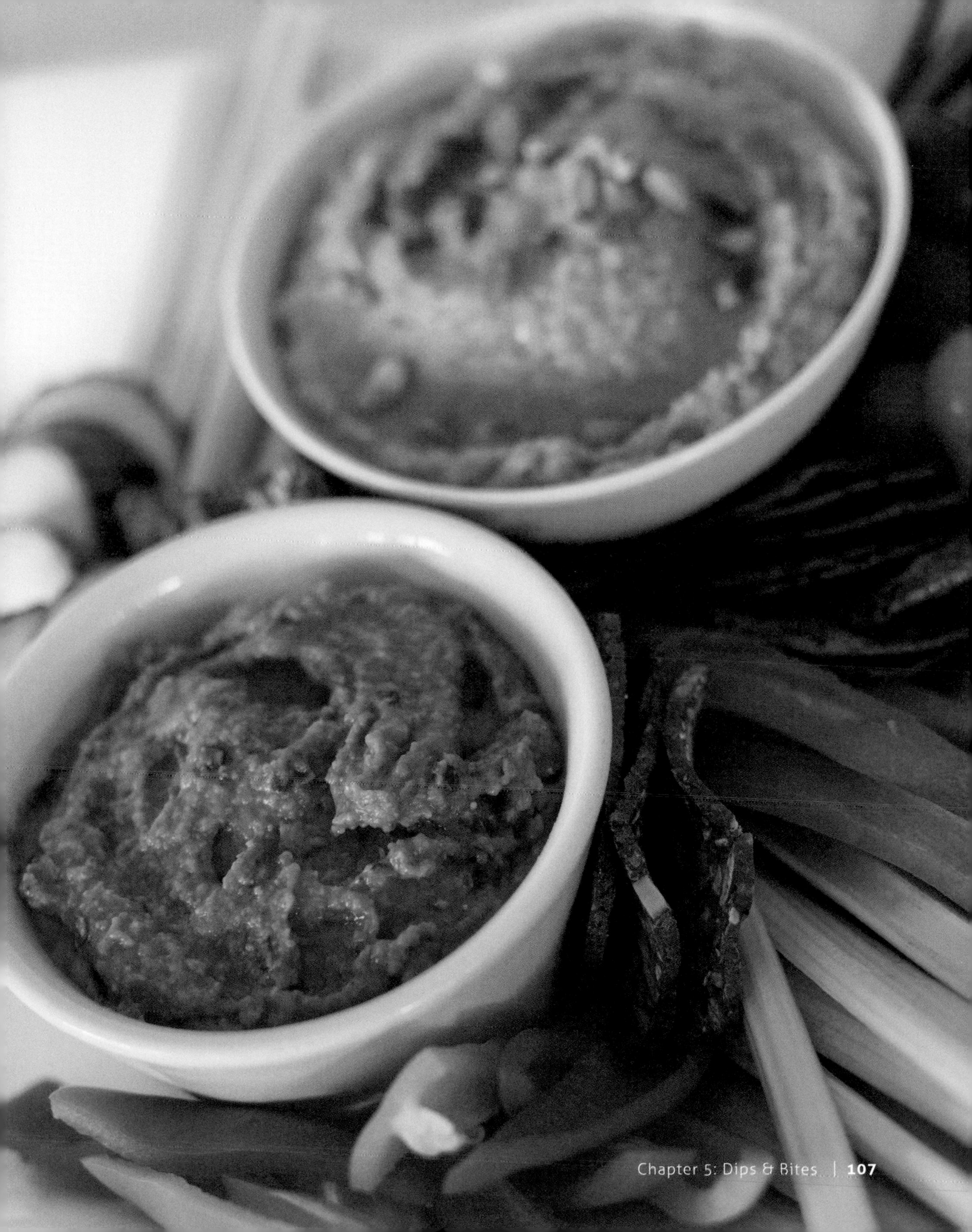

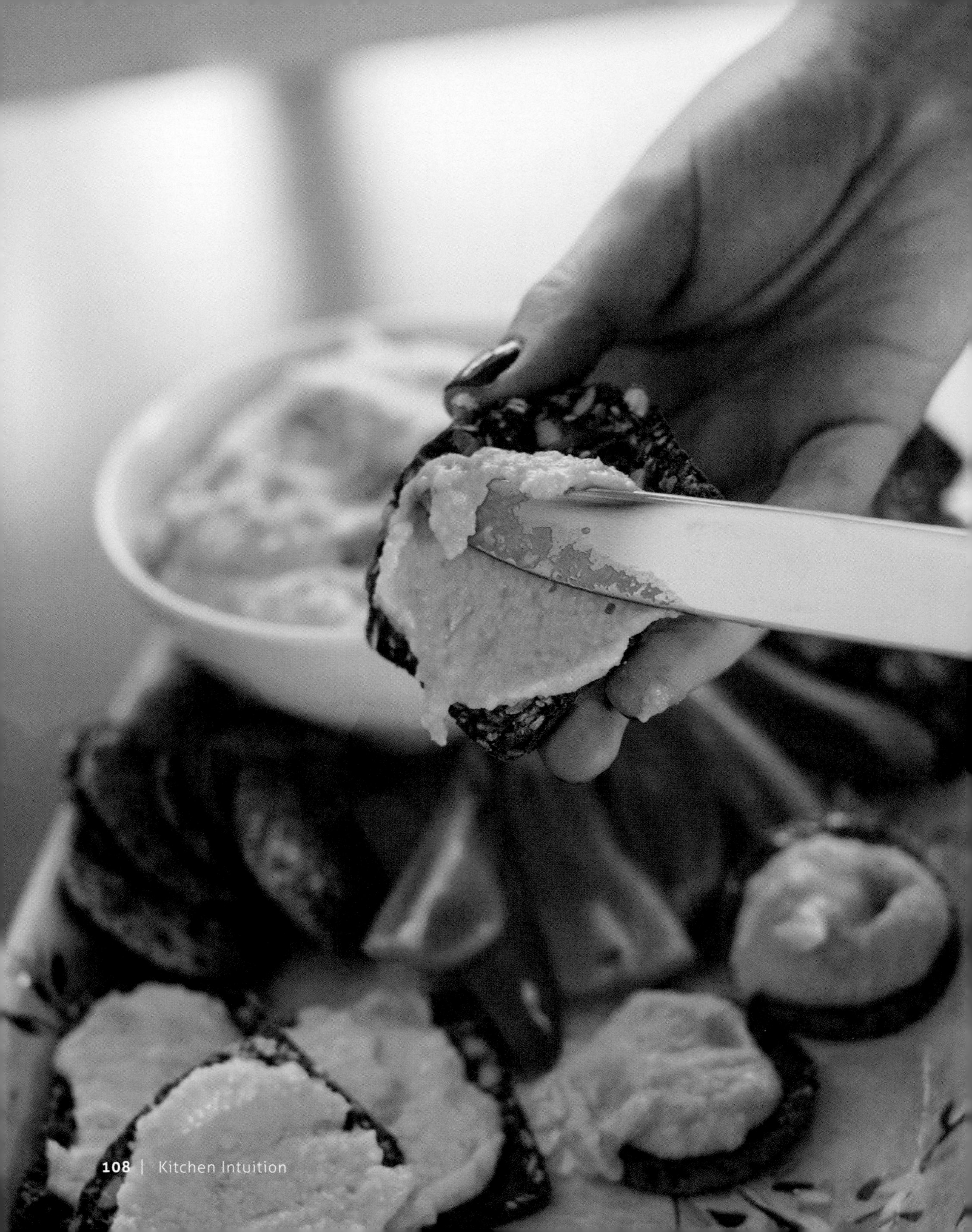

White Bean Artichoke Spread

INGREDIENTS

1 white or yellow onion, chopped

Drizzle of olive oil, for cooking and blending

1 can of white beans (cannellini)

1 can of artichoke hearts

A few cloves of garlic

1 lemon, juiced

Dash of salt

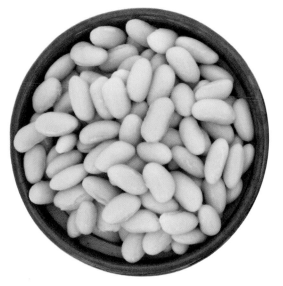

METHOD

Sauté the onion in oil for a few minutes over medium heat. In a blender or food processor, add 1 can of white beans (drained), 1 can of artichoke hearts (drained), a few cloves of garlic, the sautéed onion, olive oil, and lemon juice. Blend until smooth and salt to taste!

guacamole

The number of avocados I use in this recipe really depends on the number of guests. My general rule is half an avocado per person (unless you're a really good friend, in which case it is more like 1 or 2 avocados per person). Plus, I like leftovers, however with guac, there usually is none.

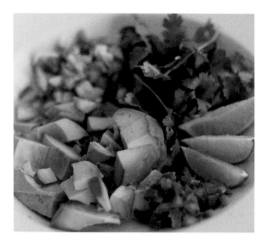

INGREDIENTS

5 avocados

1 red onion, chopped very small

1 jalapeno (seeds removed)

Cilantro (small handful of leaves only, no stems)

2 limes, juiced

Dash of salt

METHOD

Chop the onion SMALL. I don't know many people who like to eat large chunks of raw red onion. (Ok fine, I do, but most people do not.) Cut the jalapeno in half; scoop out and dispose of the seeds. Dice the jalapeno as small as you can.

(WASH YOUR HANDS. Now wash them again. I can't tell you how many times I've rubbed my eyes after cutting a jalapeno and it is no fun at all.) Pull the cilantro leaves from the stems and tear or chop them into smaller sizes.

Cut the avocados in half and remove the pits. Scoop the delicious inner green avocado flesh into a large bowl and immediately squeeze lime juice over the avocado so it doesn't turn brown. Mash up the avocado with a fork. Add in the diced onions and jalapenos, chopped cilantro, and salt. How does it taste?

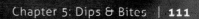

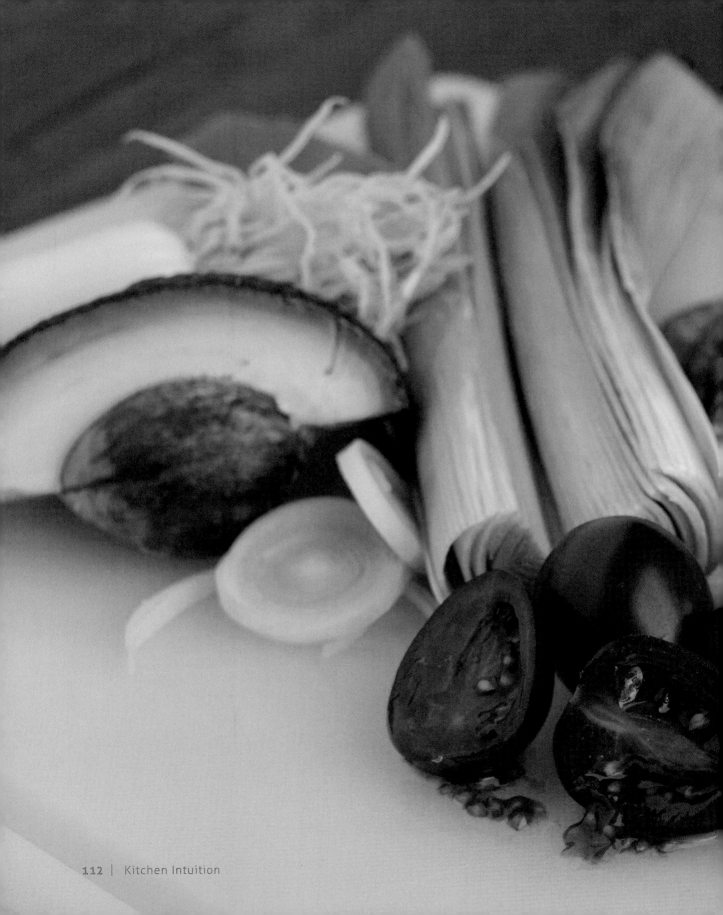

Bites

*Snacks, appetizers, and party food
(and for eating with your hands).*

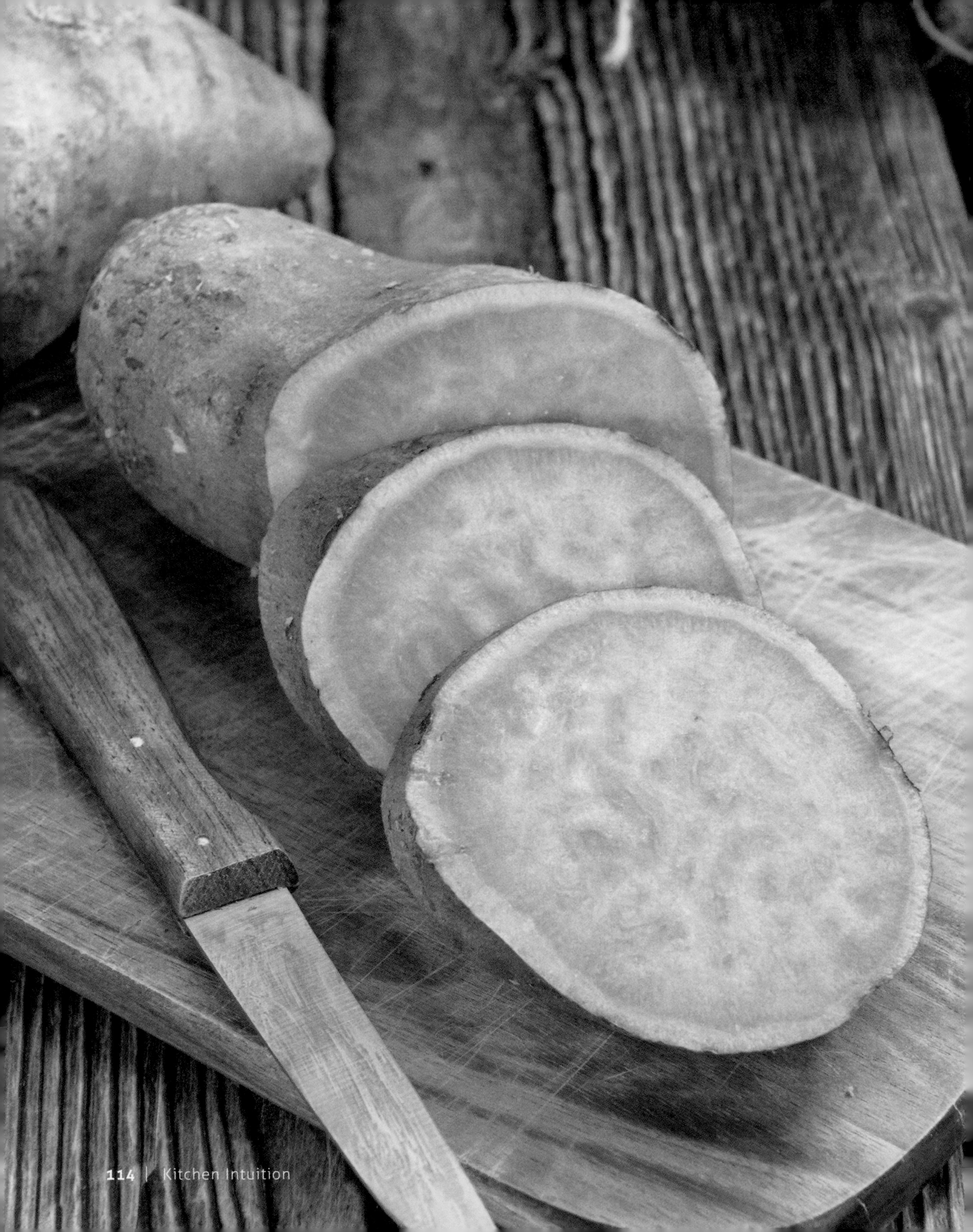

Sweet Potato, Kale, and Goat Cheese MINI TACO BITES

These little tacos were inspired by appetizers that one of my best friends and I love to make on nights before we go out. We have a glass of wine and snack on these delicious bites. She likes them a little crunchy, but I enjoy them on the softer side, which is why they became tacos!

INGREDIENTS

1 sweet potato

1 bunch of kale

Butter or oil for sautéing

Dash of garlic salt

Squeeze of lemon

3 spoonfuls of goat cheese

Drizzle of olive oil

Drizzle of honey

METHOD

Preheat the oven to 375 degrees Fahrenheit. Slice the sweet potato into rounds a ¼-inch thick. The thinner they are the crispier they'll be. Place them on a greased baking tray (or rack) and bake for 20-ish minutes, checking to see if they are cooked through and at your desired crispiness. While they are cooking, tear the leaves of kale into small pieces and sauté them in a pan with butter or oil, a pinch of garlic salt, and a squeeze of lemon. This will take a little while; low and slow is fine. You want the kale leaves to soften and cook through completely. After the sweet potato rounds have cooked and cooled enough to handle, spoon a small bit of kale onto each round. Top with goat cheese crumbles and drizzle with a tiny bit of olive oil and honey! Enjoy!

Deviled Eggs

Traditional deviled eggs usually include mustard and mayo mixed in with the yolk. I like to add things to it to make it more interesting.

INGREDIENTS

Eggs (depending on how many you want—each egg makes 2 deviled egg halves)

Dollop of mayonnaise

Dollop of mustard Small handful of crushed kale chips

Dash of curry paste/powder

Optional: chipotle peppers, lime juice

METHOD

Hard-boil the eggs by placing them in the bottom of a saucepan and covering with water. Place them on high heat until the water starts to boil. Let them boil for a minute, and then turn off the heat. Let the eggs sit covered for about 10 to12 minutes.

Rinse the eggs under cold water and peel back the shell. Slice each egg in half and carefully scoop out the yolks, preserving the cooked white part (to fill again with the deviled yolk later). Add all the yolks to a bowl and mix with a dollop of healthy mayo, mustard, the crushed kale chips, the dash of curry paste/powder, and the ingredients of your choosing. Then scoop a spoonful of the deviled yolk back into the cooked whites of the egg. Enjoy!

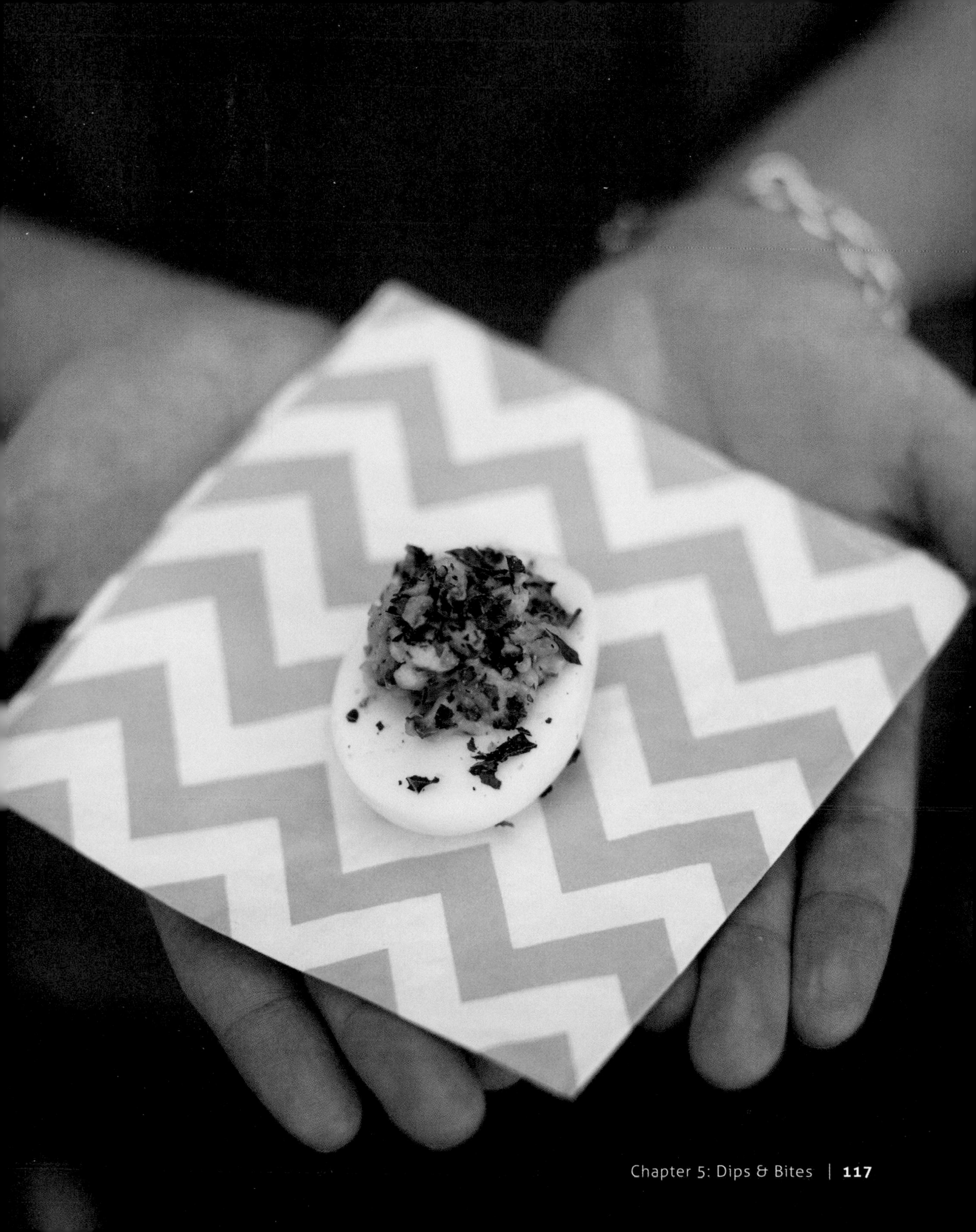

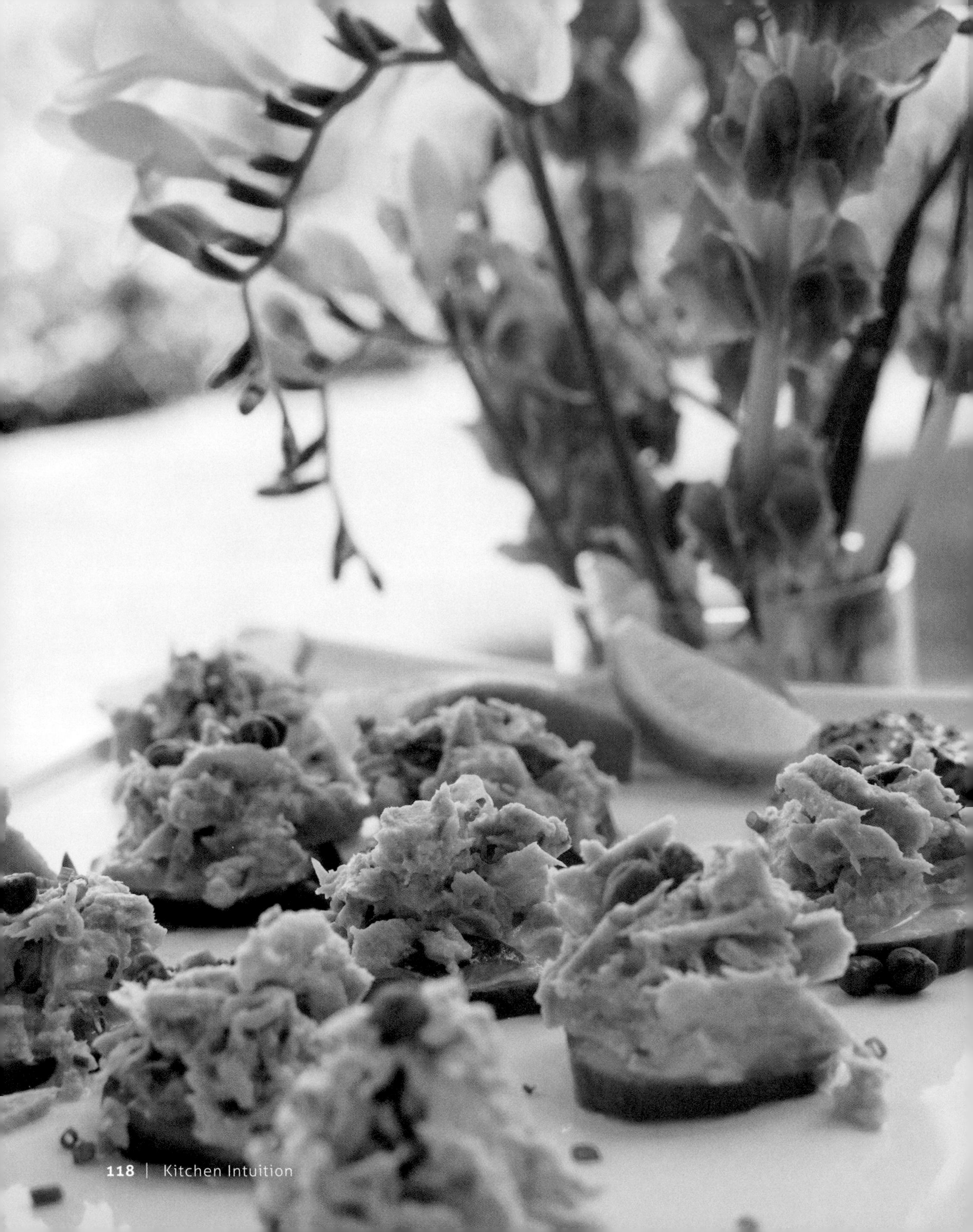

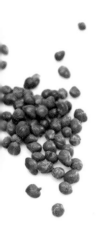

TUNA SALAD
ON
Cucumber Rounds

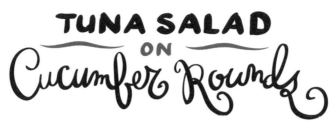

These are great for snacks or appetizers!

INGREDIENTS

¼ of a cucumber (sliced into ¼-inch rounds)

1 stalk of celery, chopped into small pieces

Handful of fresh dill, chopped

Handful of chives, chopped

1 can or jar of tuna

2 big spoonfuls of capers

A few spoonfuls of mayonnaise

1 spoonful of mustard

1 to 2 squeezes of lemon

Pinch of salt

METHOD

Slice the cucumber into ¼-inch rounds. Chop or dice the celery, dill and chives into small, easy-to-eat, pieces.

Drain the can or jar of tuna and dump the meat into a bowl for mixing. Use a fork to break up the tuna into bite-size pieces. Then mix in a few spoonfuls of mayo and one spoonful of mustard.

Add the chopped celery, dill, and chives, as well as the capers! A squeeze of lemon and a pinch of salt also will do this recipe some good. Serve the tuna salad on the cucumber rounds.

CILANTRO
Lime Wings

INGREDIENTS

Drizzle of olive oil

Small handful of cilantro (leaves only, no stems)

A few cloves of garlic, chopped

Pinch of salt

12 chicken wings

2 limes, juiced

METHOD

In a large, plastic Ziploc bag or container, mix a drizzle of olive oil, cilantro, garlic, and a pinch of salt. Add the chicken wings to the bag with the marinade and give it a shake. Its best if you let it sit for about 30 minutes.

While the chicken is marinating, preheat the oven to 350 degrees Fahrenheit. Spread the wings out on a baking sheet and bake for about 20 minutes. Flip and bake them for another 10 minutes or until golden brown and cooked through. Add the wings to a plate and squeeze lime juice over the top.

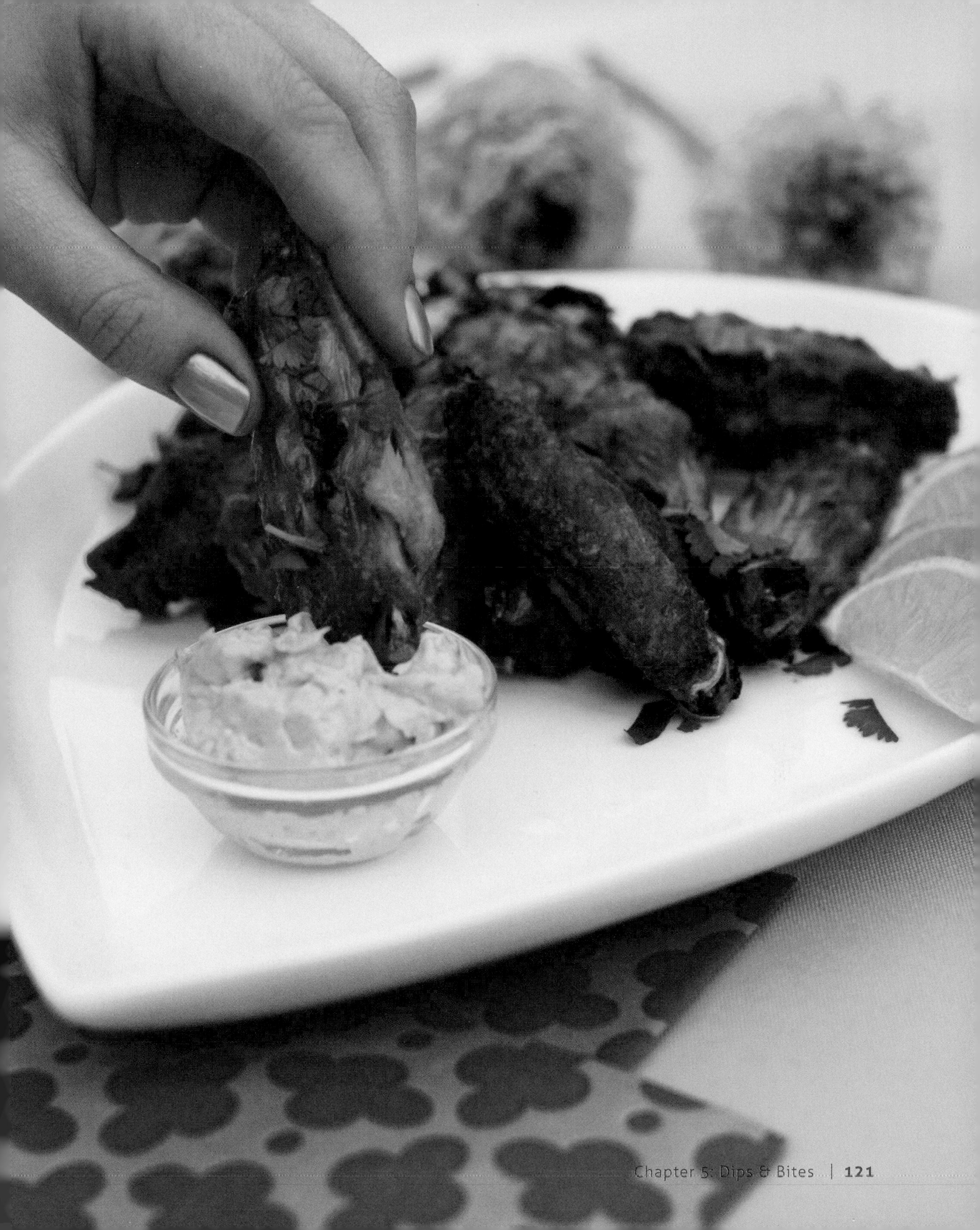

Mint Lime Watermelon

You can eat this by the pool on a hot summer day, but I also love it when I'm not feeling well. Something about the sweet and sour, salty, crunchy combination is so satisfying.

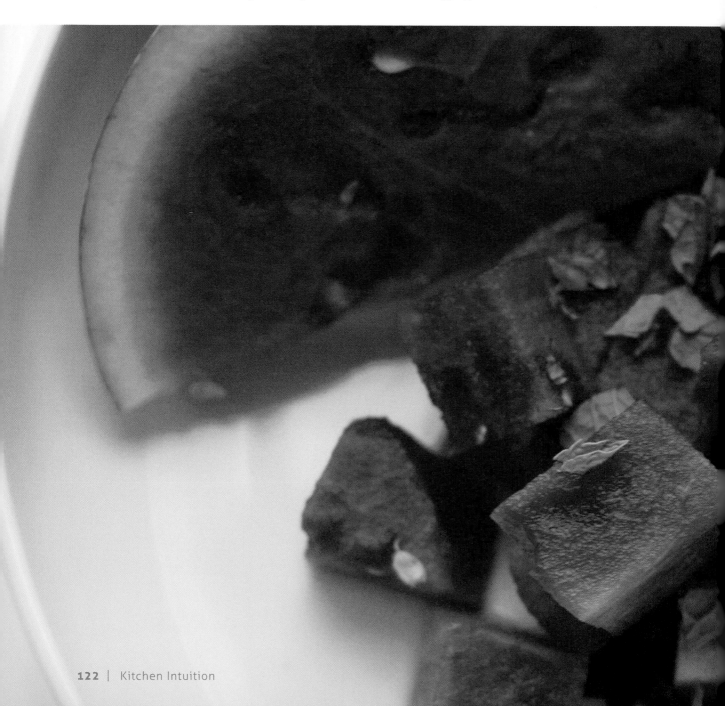

INGREDIENTS

1 watermelon (chopped)

Large handful of mint leaves

1 lime, juiced

Dash of salt

METHOD

In a large bowl, mix all the ingredients together. You simply can't mess this up. See if you can figure out a new, clever way to combine the minty, salty, sour flavor with the sweet, crunchy watermelon.

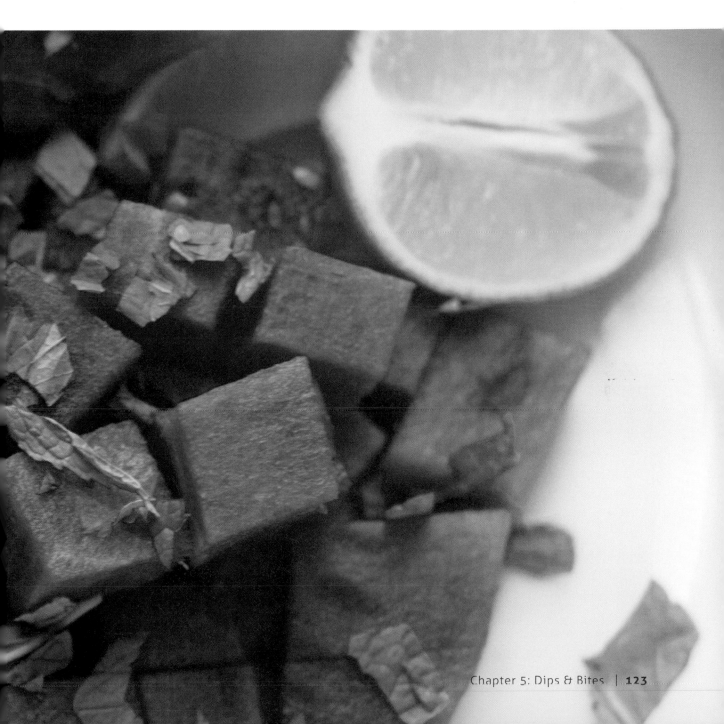

Becoming Friends with Your Kitchen and Your Food

FEEDING YOURSELF WITH LOVE

The science of nutrition is more than simply what you eat; it also encompasses how you think and feel about what you eat. The way you think about your food sends a message to your body and affects the way it is absorbed and digested. For example, if the thought of slaughtering animals for food makes you queasy about eating meat, perhaps you are more suited to a vegetarian lifestyle. Others can't get past certain smells, or textures (like with seafood dishes) to even attempt eating them. Eating is a psychological, as well as a physical experience.

Personally, I sometimes struggle with the idea of throwing my food into an appliance with a sharp blade. Blenders are loud and strike me as violent. For others, especially those who follow a raw food diet, cooking food, especially with fire is unnecessarily violent (whereas fire feels primitive, warm and comforting to me, as if it is drawing energy up from within the earth and into my food). Likewise, some people are staunchly opposed to using microwaves, while others don't mind and use them daily. How food appears in its raw form, as well as how it smells or looks as it is prepared can strongly influence our feelings and willingness to try some new dishes.

Meal preparation, like food choices, matters. In an age when convenience and speed seems to trump mindfulness in our choices, it is more important than ever to be discerning. I recently experimented by dedicating one meal each day to eating in a calm, positive environment—both inside and out. Though strange at first, I learned a few things.

For the first few days I ate alone, and became acutely aware of my tendency to distract myself; how little I chewed, how fast I ate, and how much I wanted to text friends or to watch television. I intentionally slowed down and began to pay attention. I even lit a candle. At first I found it impossible to simply sit and eat. I was overwhelmed with the need for distractions. I also noticed that I was only chewing about ten times in between bites (and that was with effort). I almost appeared to be swallowing my food whole. I also caught myself picking up another forkful of food before I was done chewing the first one! No wonder we have the tendency to overeat.

The experiment felt awkward and forced at first, but I kept reminding myself to slow down, chew, breathe, and set my fork down. Over time I came to appreciate my efforts to slow down and be mindful and to feed myself in a more relaxed and calming way. Now I try to incorporate more mindful eating habits at every meal, though it is sometimes challenging thanks to the often-hectic pace of my life. However, with practice, eating this way has become more natural and intuitive and has helped to slow my life down in more ways than one.

INTUITION DISTRACTION

One time in particular I forgot to take my own advice about cooking intuitively. In preparation for a small dinner party, I found myself in the kitchen juggling many things at once. The salmon was searing in a pan (for that crispy skin), while the water was boiling for my vegetables and wild rice was simmering away in a pot. I don't recommend doing this many things at once, but I was in a time crunch!

To lower my stress, I put on some music so that I could dance around a little as I was cooking. All of the sudden, just as I began making the miso dressing for the salmon dish, I fell out of my groove. Although wonderful, the music had taken over one of my valuable senses in the kitchen—hearing! The music drowned out the sound of the salmon searing, which tips me off that it is time to flip the fish. Nor could I hear the subtle roar of boiling water, which reminds me to throw my veggies in the pot. Then I lost track of how long the rice had been simmering. I gave myself a love tap (more like a slap), and quietly whispered, "Devyn, take your own advice: slow down and listen." This was a key turning point in realizing just how important my senses are for working in the kitchen!

DO UNTO OTHERS (EVEN YOUR FOOD)

Be nice to your food during meal preparation and your food will be nice to you. Take care of your ingredients. Give your fruits and vegetables a shower, though you don't need to soak them in water forever—just a quick rinse will suffice before they're cooked or eaten raw. Handle your fruits with care. Press gently on things like apples, peaches, avocados, or tomatoes to check for ripeness. They say that good food is made with love, and they aren't just talking about loading it up with butter (although that does help). The love and care that you put into your food preparation will be returned tenfold by the very nutrients and superior taste of such a well-crafted meal.

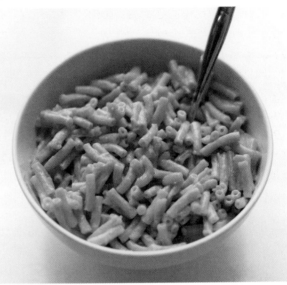

HEALTHY FOOD REBEL

I grew up in a household with a pantry stocked full of "healthier" food and snacks like Annie's organic macaroni and cheese, puffed wheat cereal, organic juices, soy milk, vegetables, whole wheat bread, and chicken nuggets made from tofu, none of which, according to me, was the "good stuff." My parents did their best to lead by example and to teach my brother and I to make healthy choices. Years later I can appreciate what they did because, let's face it, what kid knows or chooses to eat healthy food over junk food? But for a short time, their plan backfired. What I couldn't find in the pantry

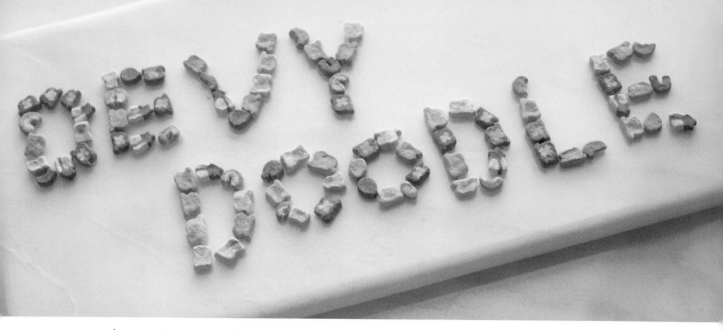

at my house, I ate at my friends' homes. I told myself, "They have all this yummy food. Their parents must love them more than mine love me." Silly, I know.

I remember having the chicken pox in kindergarten and getting to stay home from school for a week, watching cartoons while every inch of my body itched. My mom called me on her way home one day and asked what I wanted at the grocery store. She said I could have anything. *ANYTHING*? Immediately I requested Kraft Macaroni and Cheese, strawberry popsicles, and Lucky Charms cereal. This is when food became a treat, something to make me feel better.

For years, I had little to no concern for what I ate or how it was prepared. When I was old enough to make choices for myself, I responded by eating all "the good stuff" I'd missed out on those earlier years. My parents would have been mortified if they knew I was eating hot dogs, Girl Scout cookies, doughnuts, and all the Kraft Macaroni and Cheese I could get my hands on.

It is only now that I realize I was eating out of rebelliousness and for emotional comfort.

A.M. FEELINGS

Ideally, we should wake up feeling naturally energetic and ready to begin the day. I am a sucker for a good cup of Joe, but coffee is no longer something I need, but rather something I enjoy. It is important to know the difference. You may want to check in with how you're feeling in the morning to see if caffeine is something you need to wake up or just an occasional, enjoyable ritual. Rather than feeding a habit, learn to let healthy rituals nourish you. Now there's a rebellious thought.

WHEN CRAVINGS COME CALLING—FIND YOUR BALANCE

Pay attention to your cravings. You can learn a lot about your emotional and psychological health when you tune into what your body craves. This is an important tool for establishing a healthier relationship with yourself— inside and out. There is no magic formula to figuring out why you crave certain foods, but it is worth exploring what triggers you to eat, especially if the food you crave undermines rather than nourishes your health.

Some people crave sweets, while others tend to crave savory flavors. There are textural cravings like crunchy; temperature cravings like cool or hot or even spicy; and specific food cravings, like for chocolate or cheese. Pay attention to the tastes, textures and sensations that you crave. Write down what you notice about your food preferences and whether eating that food makes you feel better or worse, physically as well as emotionally.

Healthy eating doesn't mean depriving yourself of the less healthy foods that you also enjoy. Why not give yourself permission to enjoy them—on occasion? Nourish yourself with kindness by first, filling your body with nutritious food. Becoming more mindful of the food you eat and how it makes you feel will likely lead to making healthier more balanced decisions.

BROTH GOODNESS

Broth has become one of my new favorite foods. I wrote the bulk of this book during the winter months in New York. It is easy to see how vegetable, chicken, and bone broth soon became my best friends (although coffee is a close second).

Sipping broth is not only a great way to warm up, it's also a savory and filling way to hydrate and get some extra nutrients. Two of my favorite broth recipes are included in this cookbook (see pages 77–78), but don't be afraid to switch up the ingredients to suit your tastes. I keep a jug in my fridge (or freezer), and took to serving some up in my thermos as I walked down those icy Manhattan streets. These broths are also a great base for soups and for sautéing vegetables or steaming rice! In a pinch, I've sipped on broth both for dinner and breakfast!

CHEW ON THIS

If you take one thing from this book other than the cooking suggestions, digest this: CHEW YOUR FOOD. Most of us don't realize the extent to which we almost literally inhale our food. Bear in mind that just because food makes it INTO your body, doesn't mean it's doing what it was intended to do. Yes, there are acids in the stomach and a digestive tract to help break down our food, but we have TEETH for a reason.

Learning the importance of slowing down and chewing food more thoroughly has led me to a more profound appreciation of the entire eating experience. There are many obvious benefits to chewing food more thoroughly. For example, by slowing down the process of eating and simply chewing more, you end up eating less. This is because your body's feelings of satiation have a chance to kick in before you've cleaned your plate.

Chewing your food thoroughly extracts more of the flavors and nutrients of your food. It also sends signals to your stomach, triggering your digestive system to kick in. Eating slowly and chewing more consciously highlights the flavors and textures of food, making you more mindful and appreciative of your dining experience and culinary expertise!

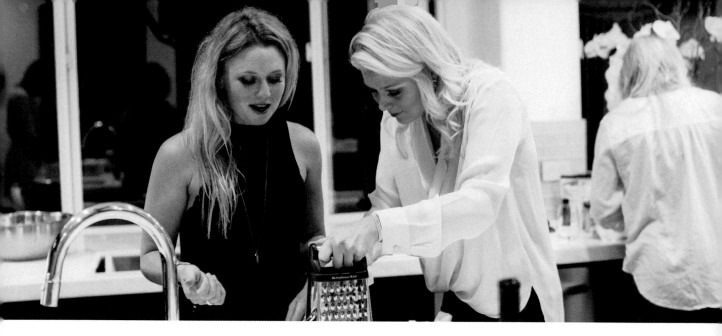

Some things to try:

- Chew each bite at least 50 times. (Easier said than done!)

- Put your fork down between each bite.

- Notice the many flavors and textures you experience as you chew.

- Eat an entire meal without your phone, television, or even a book!

- Set an intention before you eat. My favorite is: "It is my intention to eat mindfully, digest this meal with ease, absorb all the delicious nutrients, and listen to my body."

EAT IN PEACE

Your body is in a state of receiving when you eat. Not only does your body receive all the nutrients from the food you eat, it also absorbs and responds to the cues from your environment. Think of it like this: while eating lunch in a crowded mall with fluorescent lighting, amidst hundreds of crazed shoppers, with loud music blaring, your body absorbs and digests your food while in a state of stress. In contrast, your body releases far different hormones when you are eating that same lunch in a quiet café with calming music, relaxing amongst friends.

Stress hormones released in the first, more stressful scenario deliberately hampers or shuts down our digestive processes so that we can respond to perceived threats. In primitive times, the fight-or-flight response released these hormones in response to predators. In the modern world, the onslaught of loud noise, bright lights, and crowds can be stressful. This is why the second, calming environment for dining is so important. When you invite a pleasant, relaxed, outer experience *mentally* inside, you are *physically* allowing your body to digest and extract all the nutrition from your meal. So, choose dining partners and experiences that enhance your health and well-being. Be mindful that proper digestion requires a relaxed state of being, if you want to make the most of each bite.

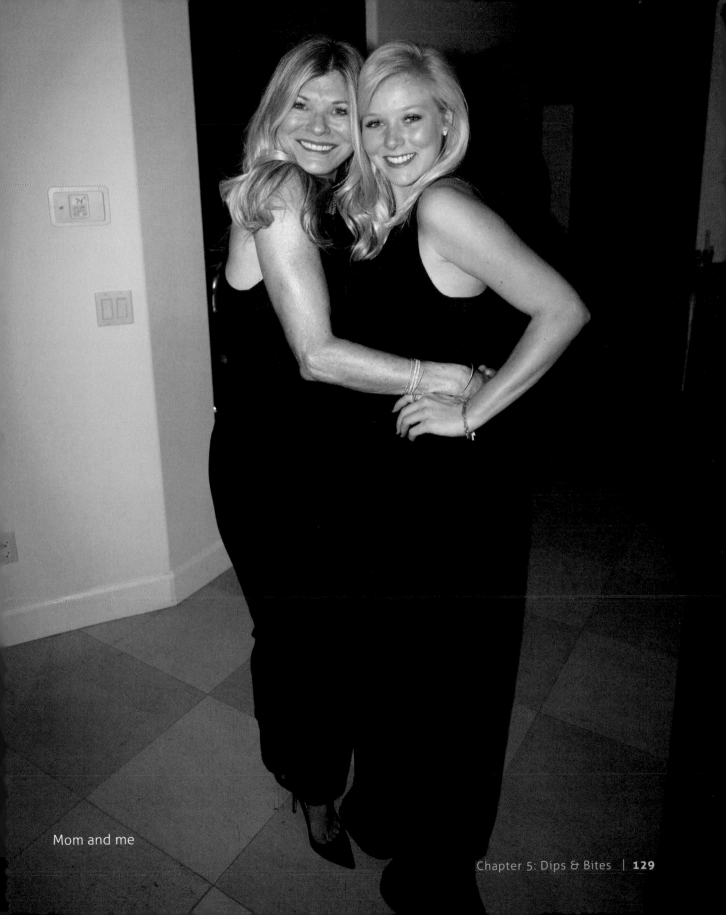

Mom and me

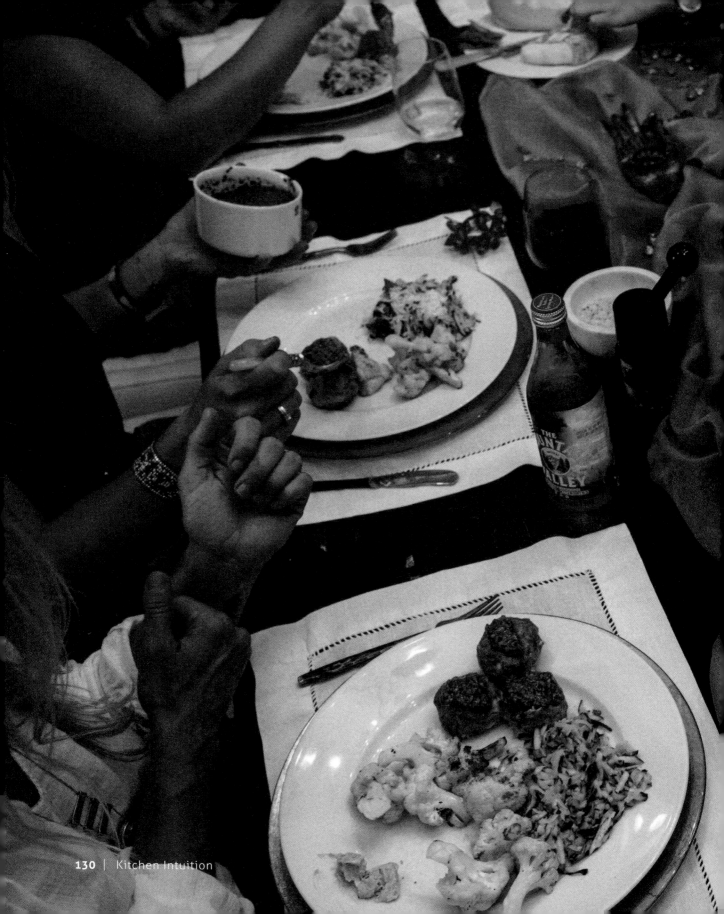

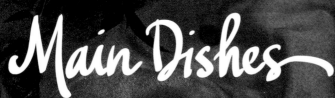

CHAPTER 6

Main Dishes

Make extra because you can always
have leftovers the next day.

Kitchen Story: Kitchen Dance

I call it the Kitchen Dance. I had just started dating M.W. and I found myself agreeing to help him cook dinner for 40 people for his birthday. We had never even been grocery shopping together. He's a guy who naturally does things last minute, so we found ourselves chaotically rushing through this culinary experience. It wasn't my normal routine, but there was something so gracefully spontaneous and efficient about it. This was a side of him, and of myself, I had never experienced.

Perhaps I didn't feel the pressure to impress anyone because, after all, these weren't my friends we were entertaining. But nor was I indifferent. Instead I felt graceful and present. Cooking with M.W. felt unusual because of how we worked so comfortably together, as if moving through the steps of a dance.

We agreed to meet at the grocery store and quickly realized that neither of us had any idea what it would be like to cook for that many people, nor how much to buy. How many onions do you think? I don't know, this many? No, two more. Ok, I trust you. It was a dance of mutual uncertainty and trust. Though he took the lead, he also graciously asked my opinion.

I had no real game plan, yet never was I more in tune with my intuition than when we were "dancing" in the kitchen. I trusted him, and myself, to work well together. Though preoccupied with cutting boards and sauté pans, I was also conscious of him next to me the entire time. We prepped the food together, marinating the steak and chopping the veggies, and then went our separate ways for a quick shower before heading back to work without missing a beat. People arrived and it was loud and chaotic. I was shaking hands, grating ginger, and blanching green beans, all at the same time.

Cooking with M.W. changed our connection with one another. Never have I felt so loved, trusted, supported, or appreciated as I did that evening. We stopped every once in a while to sneak a kiss in the pantry, acknowledging the awesomeness that was happening in the kitchen. We had at least ten people helping and offering to cut or chop things, and though hectic, somehow we all pulled it off. It was so beautifully frantic. He and I tasted each other's marinades and salad dressings, and added a pinch of this or that per one another's loving suggestions. I felt confident with him working next to me.

The dinner was an opportunity for us to shower friends with love. But sharing the meal preparation so gracefully also taught M.W. and I a new dance step—the art of letting go and trusting.

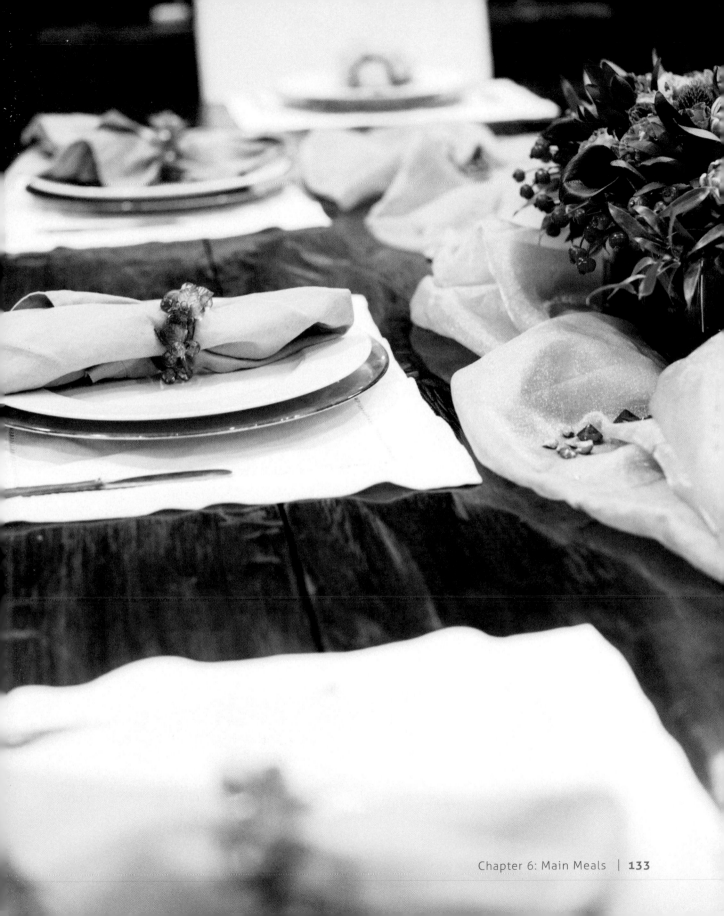

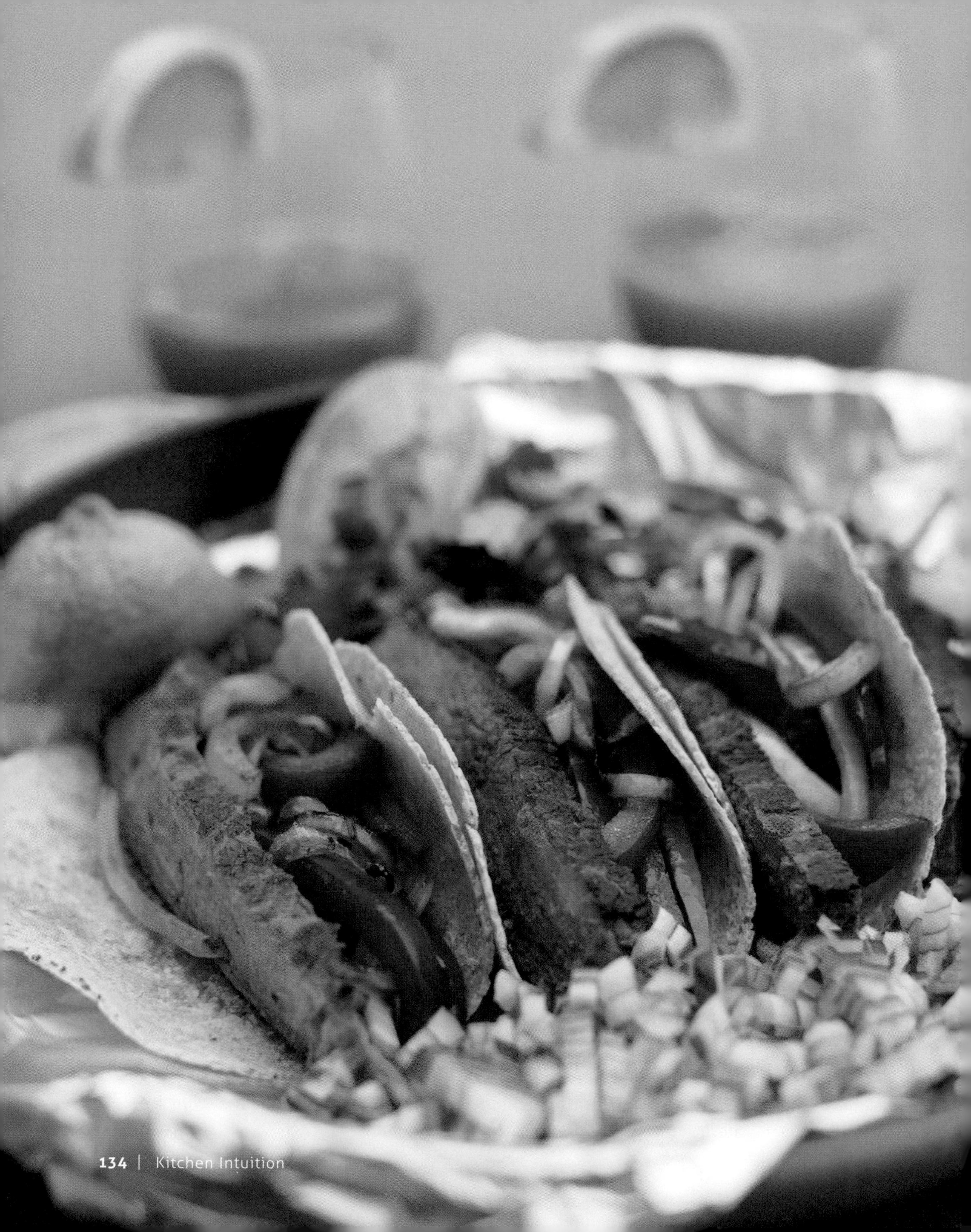

Fajita Tacos

INGREDIENTS

¼ to ½ pound of steak per person (any kind will work, but I prefer hanger or flank steak)

Spices for the steak—a few dashes each of:

cumin

paprika

onion powder

chili powder

salt

1 or 2 bell peppers (red, orange, or yellow)

1 onion, sliced lengthwise into thin strips

Drizzle of olive oil, for cooking

Tortillas (1 to 2 per person—corn, flour, or homemade)

Small handful of cilantro (leaves only, no stems)

Hot sauce to taste

Optional: chopped avocados (again, not optional in my home); grated cheese (recommend cheddar or Monterey Jack)

METHOD

Season your steak by shaking a few dashes of each spice onto both sides of your steak. Get your hands dirty and give it a good rub. A massage even. Slice your bell peppers into long, thin strips. Slice up your onion in a similar shape to the bell peppers so they cook evenly together.

In a hot skillet with a drizzle of oil, add your steak! Cook on medium-high for a few minutes on each side until cooked to your liking, and then set it aside to rest. (Once you remove it from the heat, it will continue to cook through for a few more minutes.)

In the same pan, add a bit more oil, the peppers, and the onions. Stir them around for a few minutes until they are slightly browned on either side. Let the veggies soak up the flavors from the steak.

After the steak has had a chance to rest for at least 5 minutes, thinly slice the meat against the grain.

Gently warm the tortillas by setting them on a baking sheet in the oven on a low temperature (under 300 degrees Fahrenheit). Keep an eye on them because they toast up quickly. (You can also warm tortillas on a skillet over low heat.)

Wash the cilantro and pull the leaves from the stems. If you like, chop an avocado into bite-size pieces.

Assemble your fajita tacos with your cooked ingredients. Then add the cilantro, avocados, and hot sauce. Even grated cheese if you wish! YUM!

This was inspired by my "aunt's" amazing potato chip chicken recipe. I experimented and figured out that I could use just about anything crunchy and salty to make this work. Make extra because this is great for leftovers.

INGREDIENTS

A few eggs (about 1 egg per 2 chicken breasts)

2 or 3 handfuls of chips (I use taro root chips and beet chips, but I encourage experimenting)

1 pound of boneless, skinless chicken breasts (you can slice them into long, thin chicken tender strips)

Dash of salt and pepper

Spoonful of ghee, for cooking

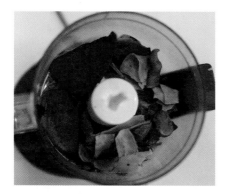 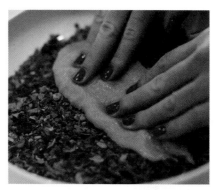

METHOD

Beat the eggs in a bowl and set aside.

Pour the chips (or crackers) into a resealable plastic bag, seal closed, and then use anything heavy to pound the chips into a crunchy powder. (A spatula or rolling pin can be fun to use.) Pour the crushed chips onto a large plate or bowl.

Lightly season the chicken with salt and pepper one breast at a time. Then dip the chicken into the beaten egg mixture. Next dredge the chicken onto the plate of crushed chip crumbs. Cover the chicken as best as you can with the crunchy chip goodness.

Preheat a pan with a spoonful of ghee and cook the chicken breasts. (You can also bake them in an oven at 375 degrees Fahrenheit for 40 minutes, or until the chicken is no longer pink in the middle.)

I love using this leftover chicken in a wrap or chopped up on a salad the next day! It isn't as crunchy as a leftover, but it still has a nice flavor that is different from regular grilled chicken.

ANY CHIP
Chicken

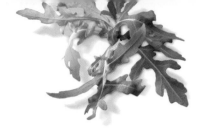

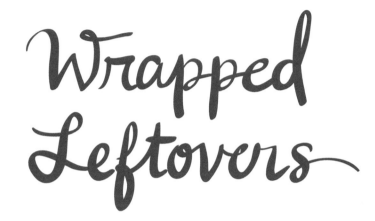

Wrapped Leftovers

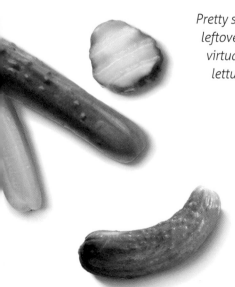

Pretty self-explanatory, right? Pictured here is a store-bought coconut wrap filled with leftover **Any Chip Chicken** *(see recipe on page 136) and some veggies! You can use virtually any of the recipes in this cookbook as a wrapped leftover the next day. I add lettuce, avocado, and pickles to almost anything and call it a meal!*

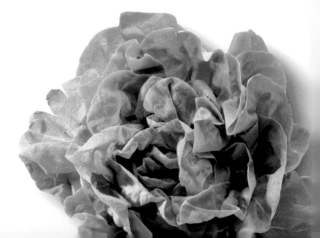

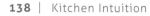

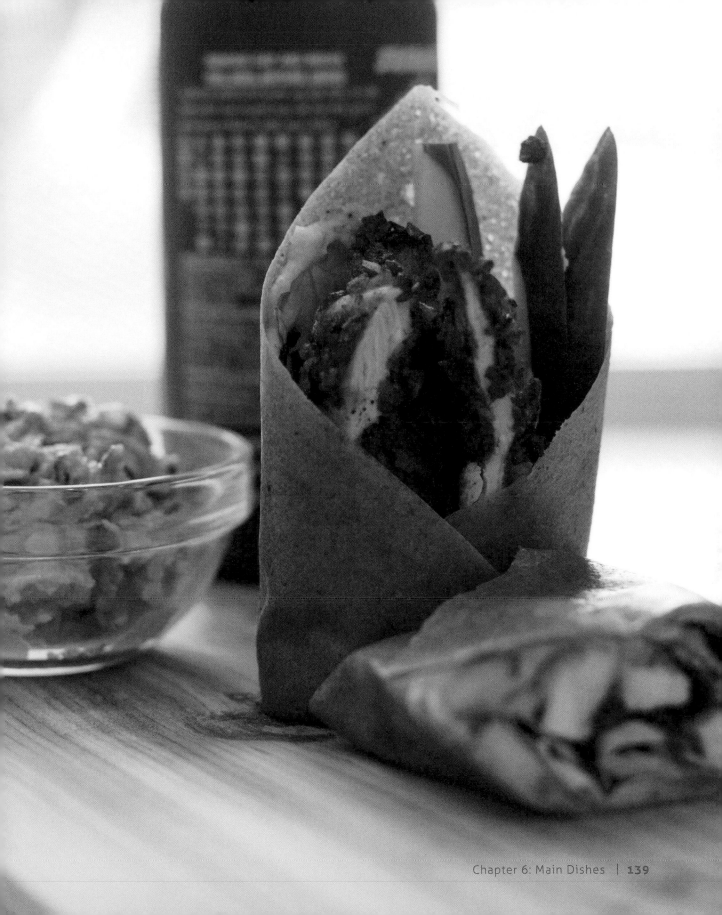

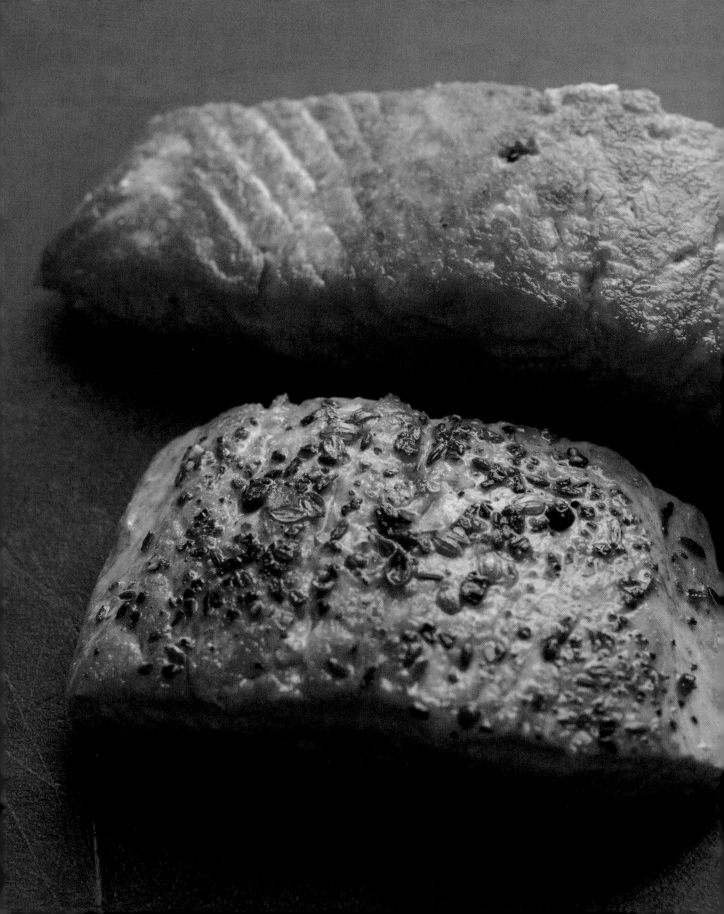

Salmon - THE BASICS

Always buy good quality fish. I buy from a fish market or farmers' market whenever possible, and I usually steer away from buying it frozen. Here's to keeping it simple and fresh.

INGREDIENTS

1 6-ounce piece of deboned, skinned salmon

Dash of salt

Drizzle of oil or pat of butter for cooking

METHOD

Lightly salt both sides of the salmon.

Place the salmon in a preheated and oiled or buttered pan. Sear each side of the fish on high heat for a few minutes.

You can tell how cooked the fish is by looking at the sides of the meat. Once it looks done halfway up, flip it over and sear the other side for a minute or two.

COOKING TIP

This works with any fish, and I encourage you to experiment with cooking different types. Salmon is my favorite right now, but it changes all the time. Although there are many other ways to cook fish, the simplest and most reliable way I found is to lightly season and cook it in a pan with some butter, ghee, or oil.

TASTE TIP

You can season your fish with just about any flavors you like, and I encourage you to experiment with herbs and spices! (Although sometimes less is more, and I have never been disappointed with this lightly salted, seared salmon.) I can add it to anything—a salad or any veggie sides, in wraps for lunch, or even in sandwiches. Enjoy!

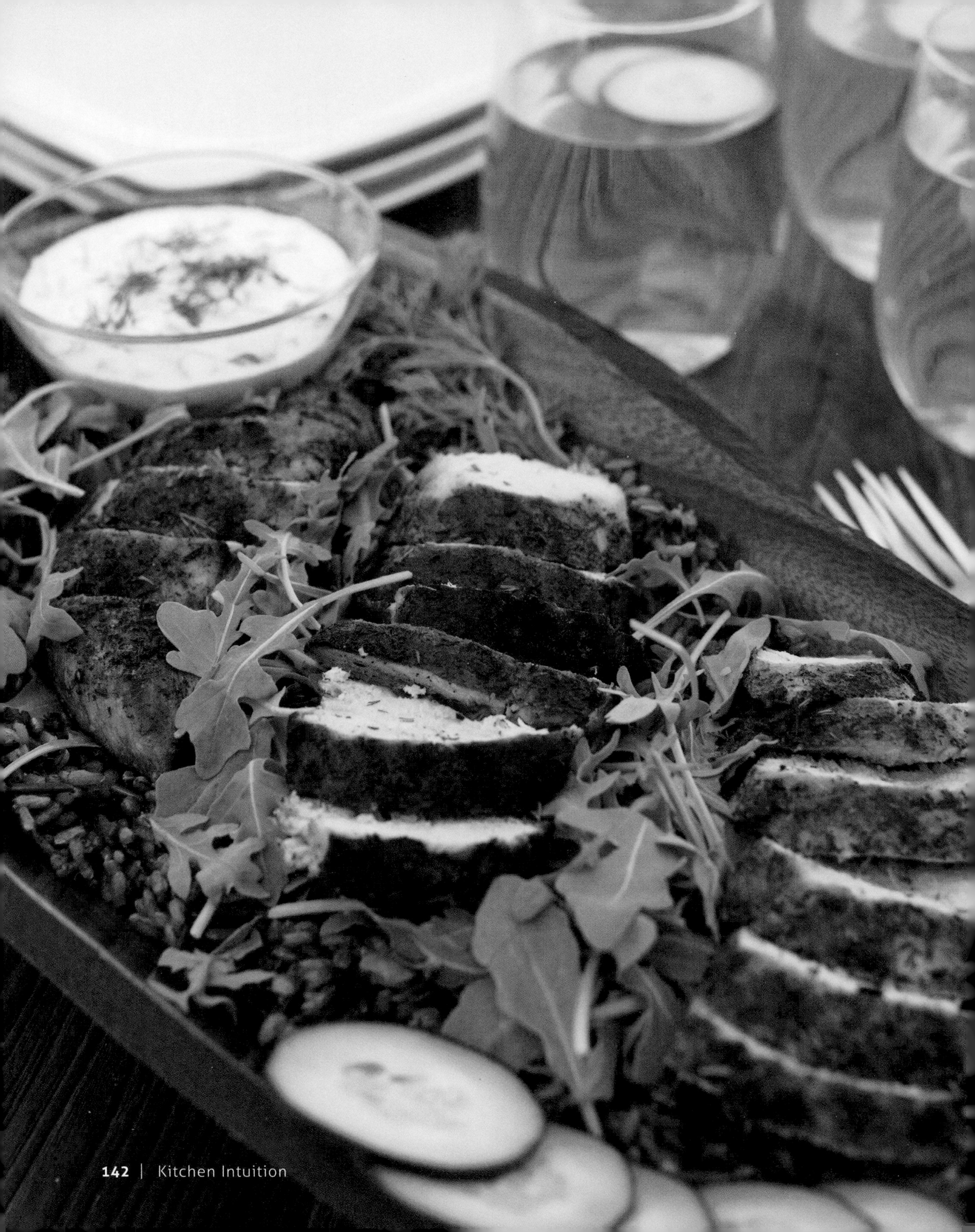

Chicken with Wild Rice and Arugula

INGREDIENTS

½ to 1 cup of wild rice (per serving)

8 ounces of boneless chicken breasts (per person)

Dash of salt and pepper

A few spoonfuls of Greek yogurt

A few limes, juiced

Drizzle of olive oil

Handful of arugula

½ cucumber, diced small or grated

Handful of fresh dill leaves

1 garlic clove, diced small

METHOD

Cook the wild rice according to the package. As the rice is cooking, salt and pepper both sides of the chicken breasts and cook them on the grill or in a lightly oiled, preheated pan on high for a few minutes. Cook on both sides until the chicken is no longer pink in the middle.

In a small bowl, mix a few heaping spoonfuls of Greek yogurt with the juice of a few limes and a drizzle of olive oil. In another medium bowl, add the arugula, cucumber, dill, garlic and some salt. Stir and taste.

When the rice has cooled and the chicken is done, add to the bowl of vegetables, mix, and top with the sauce!

Asian Turkey Meatballs
with Bok Choy

INGREDIENTS

2 shallots (or half an onion), chopped

Ginger, minced (small handful of the root)

3 to 4 garlic cloves

½ pound of ground turkey

3 green onions, chopped

A few pinches of salt

2 eggs

Drizzle of sesame oil, for cooking

Dash of soy sauce

Handful of bok choy, chopped

METHOD

Chop up 2 shallots or half an onion. Mince a small handful of ginger as fine as you can. Mince 3 or 4 garlic cloves as fine as you can.

In a bowl, mix together the ground turkey, green onions, shallots, garlic, ginger, and a few pinches of salt. Crack and beat 2 eggs and then add into the mixture. Get your hands dirty by forming the turkey mixture into meatballs. Do not overmix.

In a hot pan, drizzle some sesame oil and place the meatballs in a circle. You want to hear the meatballs sizzle when you place them in the pan. Cook the meatballs for a few minutes on each side, rotating them as you go. When they feel firm to the touch, cut into one and make sure the meat looks cooked through and the juices run clear. When done, set the meatballs aside on a plate to cool.

In the same pan, sauté some bok choy with sesame oil, soy sauce, and a pinch of salt. Serve the bok choy as a side to the meatballs.

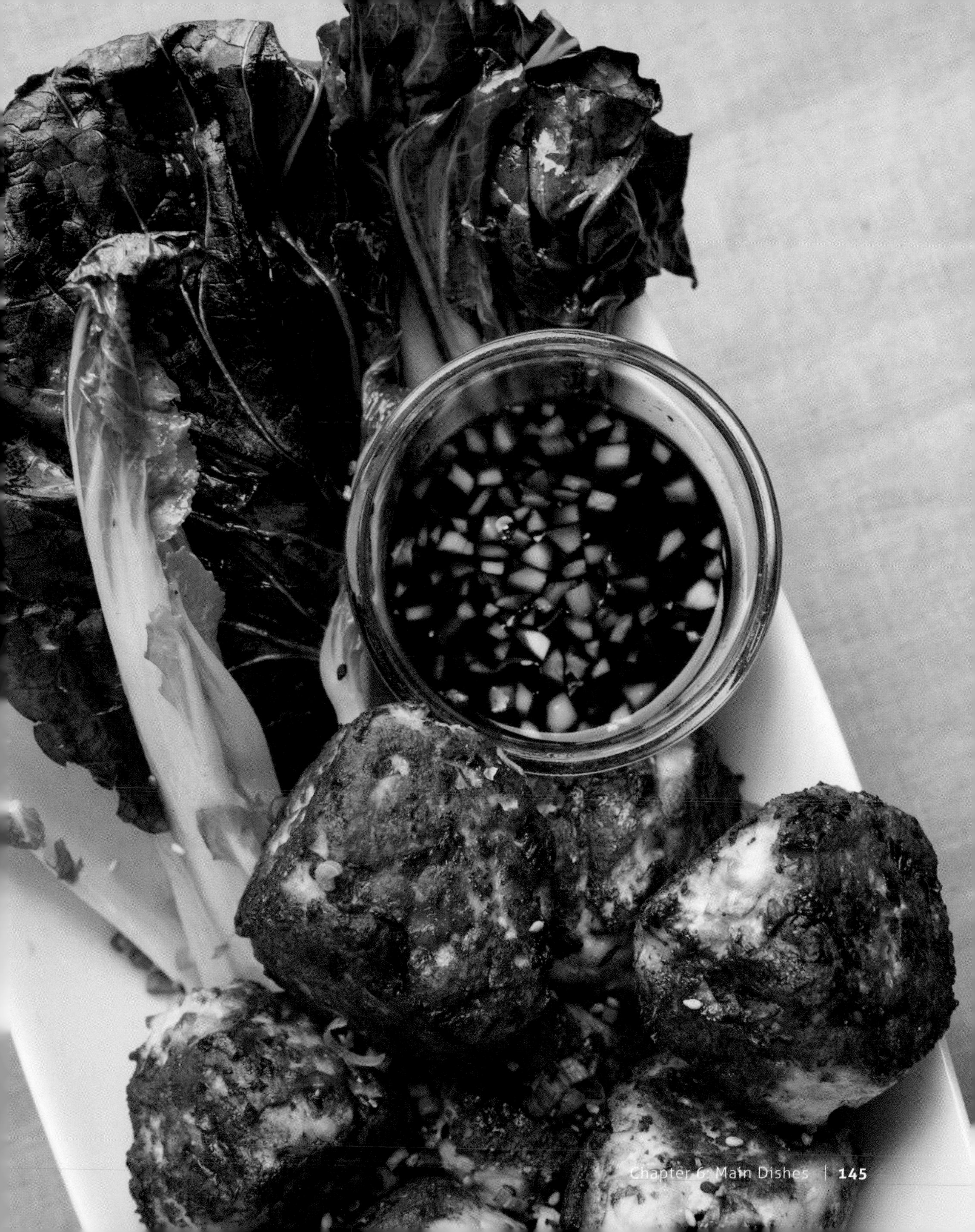

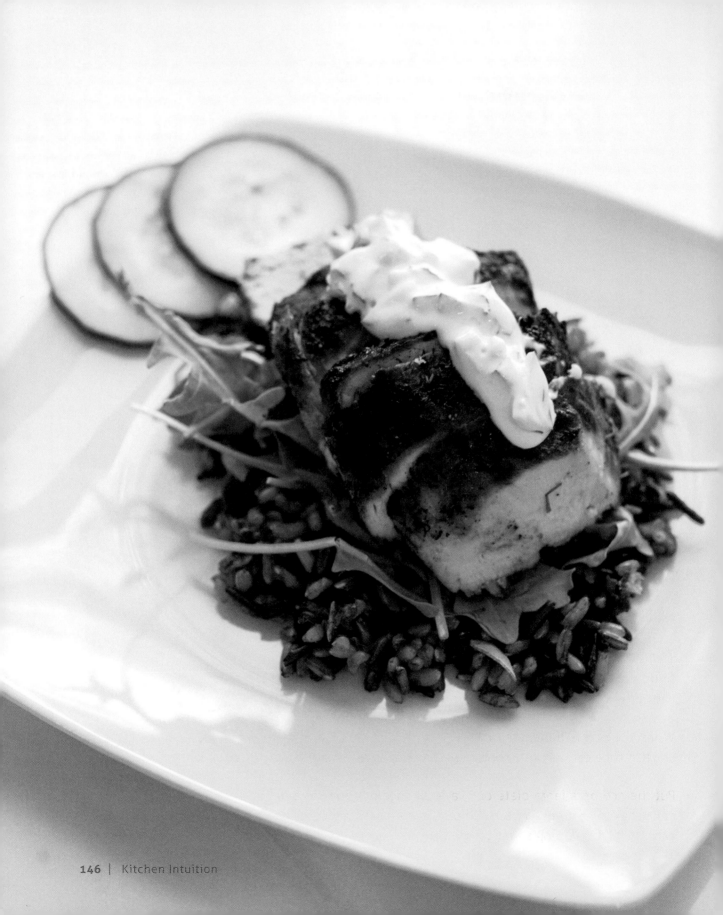

Grilled Herb Chicken
WITH
Wild Rice, Arugula, and Tzatziki

INGREDIENTS

1 cup of wild or brown rice

Chicken (1 breast or thigh per person)

Ghee, coconut oil or butter for cooking

Handful of arugula

Optional spices for chicken: salt, pepper, garlic powder, oregano, or cumin

For the Tzatziki:

1 cup of Greek yogurt

½ cucumber

Handful of mint leaves

1 lime, juice and zest

METHOD

Prepare the rice as directed on the package. (It usually takes a while so you might want to start on this first.)

Flavor the chicken however you like—try salt, pepper, garlic powder, oregano, or cumin.

Once you have spiced up the chicken (on both sides), cook it on a grill or sear it in a pan. Make sure whatever surface you are cooking on is hot before setting the chicken on it. This will give it a nice crispy texture on the outside. Cook for a few minutes on each side or until the juices inside are clear and the chicken is firm to the touch. Overcooking chicken isn't the worst thing in the world, but undercooking it can be.

To make the tzatziki:

Chop up about half a small cucumber and some mint leaves. Zest one lime. Mix it all together with Greek yogurt and the juice of one or two limes.

When the rice is done, you may want to add some of the same spices you used to flavor the chicken. Rice can be pretty boring on its own, but adding spices is an easy way to flavor it up.

Put the rice on a large plate or in a bowl, mix in a few large handfuls of arugula, and slice the chicken on top. You can pour the tzatziki sauce over the chicken and mix it all together, or you can use it as a dipping sauce on the side, whichever you prefer.

Shakshuka

Shakshuka is a delicious Middle Eastern and North African egg and vegetable dish. It is great to serve for breakfast or brunch or even a weeknight dinner. Though the version of the recipe below includes sausage, Shakshuka can also be a great meatless option to serve your vegetarian family and friends, as long as they eat eggs!

INGREDIENTS

1 to 2 chicken sausages or chorizo (per person)

Drizzle of coconut or avocado oil or butter for cooking

1 onion

1 bell pepper (I prefer red, orange, or yellow ones for this recipe)

3 to 5 cloves of garlic, chopped

Pinch of the following:

paprika

cumin

cayenne pepper

salt

2 cans of chopped tomatoes

4 eggs

Handful of feta cheese (or goat cheese, crumbled although any cheese will be delicious)

Small handful of cilantro leaves, chopped (no stems)

METHOD

If you are using uncooked chicken sausage, the first step is to cut the casing or skin off and then crumble the pieces of sausage into a preheated, lightly oiled pan on medium heat. (If the sausage is already cooked, then add it in later to reheat with the vegetables.)

Cut up the onion and bell pepper into medium to large pieces or slices. On medium heat, add some butter or oil to a large pan and sauté the onions and peppers until they are soft and golden. (A crunchy texture is not recommended for this recipe.) Add the precooked sausage to the vegetables to reheat it.

While the pan of vegetables and sausage cook, add in 3 to 5 cloves of chopped garlic (depending on how much you like). It is best to add the garlic to the vegetables and sausage during the last few minutes of sautéing.

Next, add the spices to the garlic, vegetables, and sausage. Experiment for yourself with the paprika, cumin, cayenne pepper (rather spicy), and salt. (I tend to use big pinches.) Next, add the canned tomatoes. Let everything cook on low heat for another couple of minutes or until the sauce starts to thicken.

Using the back of a spoon, make 4 small holes in your mixture. (These will serve as little nests for the eggs to cook in.) Carefully crack one egg at a time, and slowly pour it into the nests/holes that you created (one egg per nest/hole). Sprinkle the crumbled or grated cheese all over the pan and cover with a tight lid for a few more minutes or until the eggs are cooked to your liking.

Salmon Burgers

You can make these burgers using most types of fish. Tuna, halibut, and snapper are just the ones I've tried. Buy fish from a reliable fish or farmers' market. When possible, choose wild-caught fish and ask to have the skin removed for easier preparation.

INGREDIENTS

1 to 2 green onions, chopped

½ white or yellow onion

Small handful of dill, chopped (preferably fresh)

1 pound of salmon (or one of the fish mentioned above)

1 egg

Handful of almond flour (or small handful of bread crumbs or cooked quinoa—as binder for the burgers)

A few pinches of salt

Oil for cooking (coconut or olive oil, butter, or ghee)

Optional: capers

METHOD

Chop the green onion as fine as you can into little tiny rounds until you have a handful. Dice the half onion.

Chop the fresh dill, though you can also use your hands to tear off the leaves.

Remove the skin from the fish if it isn't already done, and chop the fish into tiny pieces. Lay out the chopped fish onto a flat surface and then run your knife through it to continue chopping into smaller bits, almost like minced meat. (You want the pieces small enough so that they don't break apart in the pan. You want them to become ONE again.)

In a large bowl, mix together the minced fish, onions, egg, and a small handful of almond flour. Add a few pinches of salt, and a small handful of fresh dill (or a spoonful, if dried).

Preheat an oiled pan (using coconut or olive oil, butter, or ghee) over medium heat. Form the salmon mixture into 4 patties and place into the pan, cooking for a few minutes on each side until they are golden brown and cooked through to your preference.

COOKING TIP

I usually eat these without a bun because they are delicious on their own. You can use lettuce as a wrap or a couple lightly roasted large portabella mushrooms as a "bun." Or you can just use a regular bun! These are fantastic served with mustard, pesto, or aioli! (See Pesto Chimichurri recipe on page 105.)

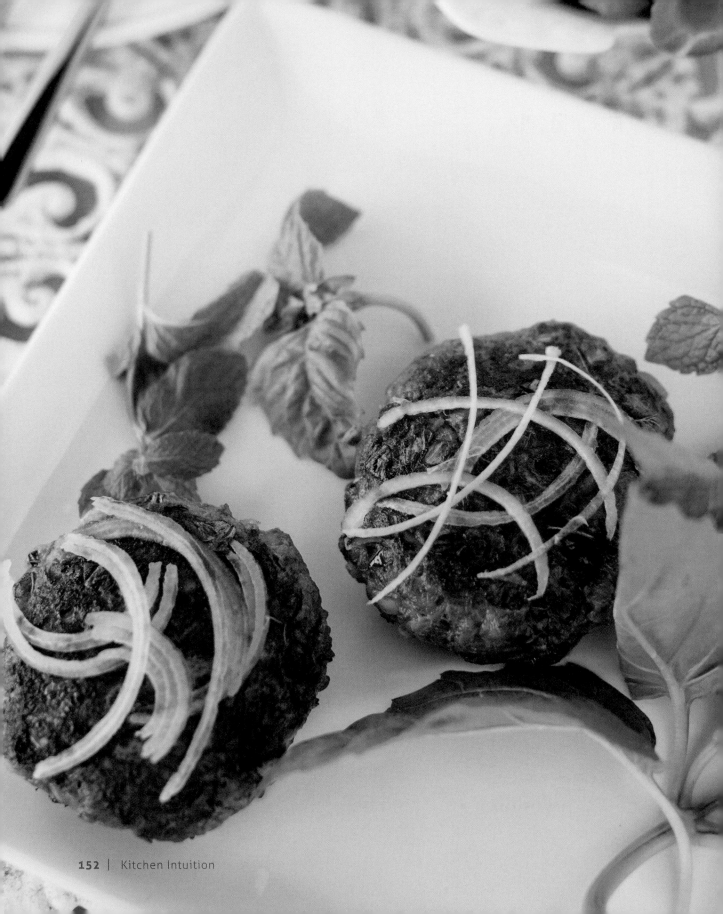

Lamb Burgers

Because sometimes I don't wanna eat beef. Lamb coming right up!

INGREDIENTS

1 pound of ground lamb

1 onion, diced

A few mint leaves, chopped

Dash of oregano

Big spoonful of mustard

Small pinch of crushed red pepper flakes

Oil for cooking (coconut oil, butter, or ghee)

Sprinkle of salt

METHOD

Pull apart the ground lamb and put into a mixing bowl. Dice the onion pretty small, and chop up a few mint leaves. Add the onion, mint leaves, a dash of oregano, a big spoonful of mustard, and a small pinch of red pepper flakes into the bowl with the lamb. Get your hands dirty by mixing all the ingredients together.

Preheat an oiled pan (using coconut oil, butter, or ghee to coat it) over medium-high heat. Form the meat mixture into patties, sprinkling both sides with salt. When the pan is hot, place the burgers in and cook both sides for a few minutes each or until cooked through to your liking!

Chicken Salad Sandwich

Leftover chicken breasts make great chicken salad!
Get your hands dirty and shred the chicken with your fingers.

INGREDIENTS

Several leftover (cooked)
chicken breasts

1 celery stalk, chopped

½ onion, chopped

Herbs of your choice (chopped, if fresh,
or a dash, if dried; try mint, dill, thyme,
chives, or cilantro)

A few spoonfuls of mayonnaise

1 spoonful of mustard

Bread slices or lettuce leaves or a wrap

Optional: capers

METHOD

Shred the chicken or chop into small bite-size pieces. Put into a mixing bowl with the chopped celery, onion, and herbs. Toss in a few dollops of mayonnaise and one dollop of mustard (or your preference). Mix all ingredients together. If you would like to, add capers. Use bread to make a sandwich, or try lettuce leaves or wraps to eat your leftover chicken salad.

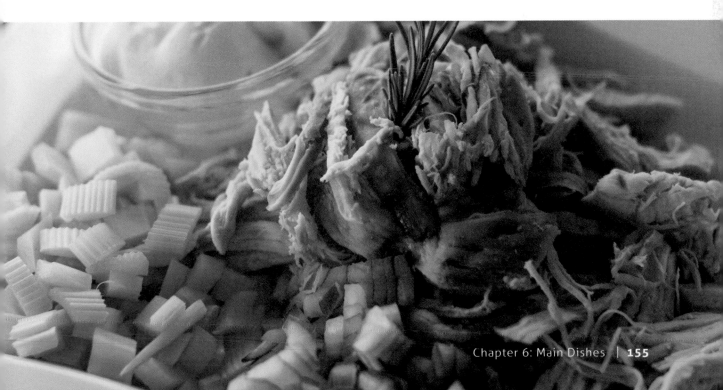

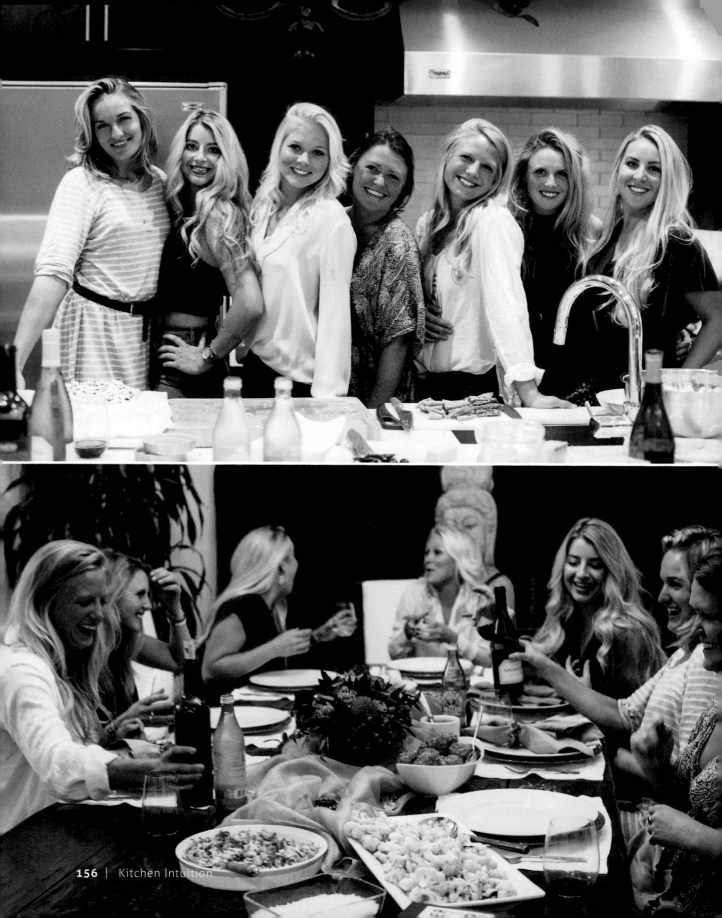

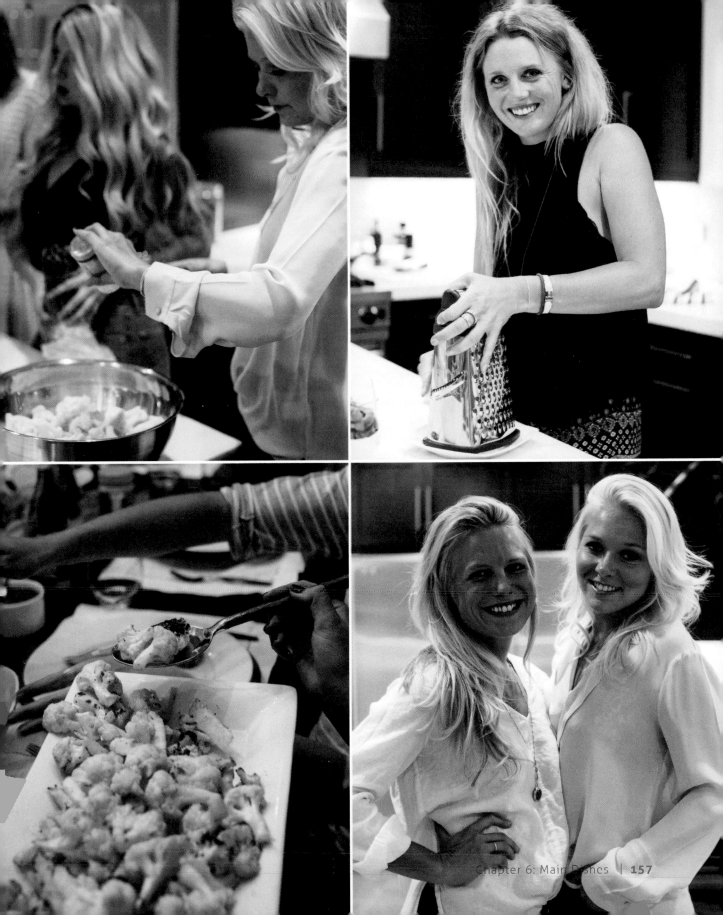

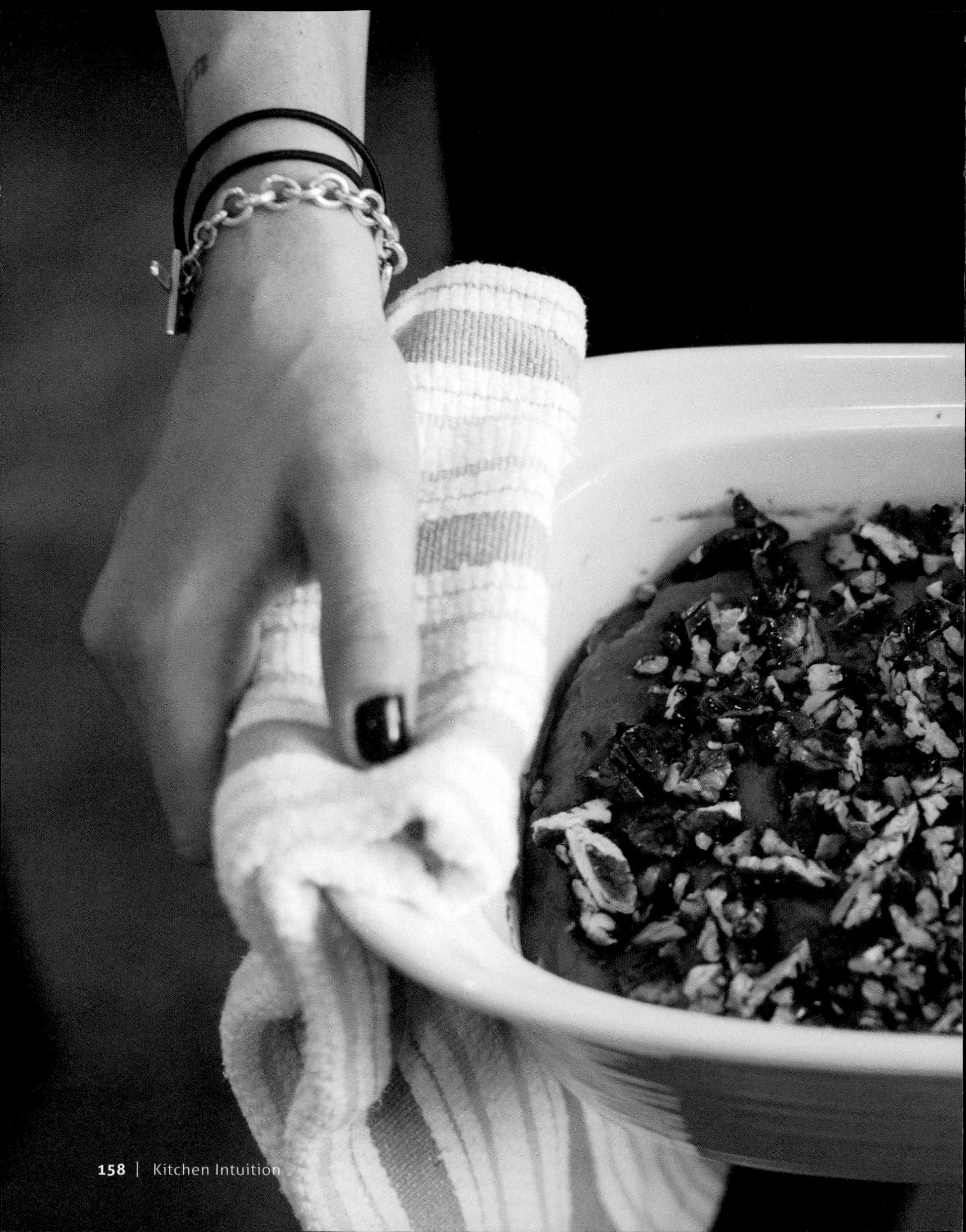

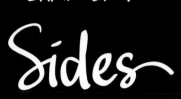

CHAPTER 7:

Sides

Sides are a great addition to main dishes, but they are often good as a standalone meal or as leftovers for lunch.

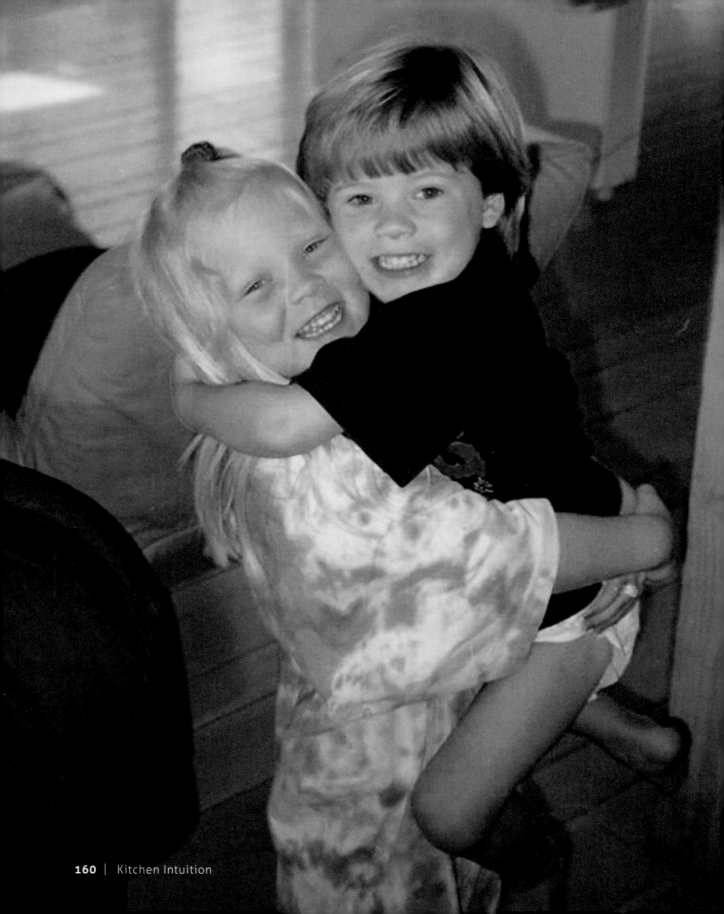

Kitchen Story: My Brother, My Teacher

Families often have a difficult time cooking and eating together because of picky eaters and varying dietary restrictions. Nowhere is this more apparent than in my family, where each person's individual taste has diverged and evolved over the years. My parents are both in peak physical condition, which sets a high bar, and to be fair, who wouldn't want to follow in their footsteps? To their credit, they never pressured me to eat a certain way. I had to forge my own path to healthy eating. It took years to give myself permission to experiment with my own diet and to figure out what feels best for me. I am still learning.

This personal struggle is one of the many reasons I admire my brother. I have learned that making healthy food choices was difficult for him as well. He silently struggled with what works for him and what he thought he "should" be eating. What I realized recently is that Kyle also had to learn to listen to his own intuition. As a vegetarian, Kyle has been going against the varying dietary theories of our family. But he is happy, healthy, and strong and feels good about his own food choices.

As a young college guy growing into himself both physically and mentally, I watched Kyle battle with the decision to stay a vegetarian. After all, his family and friends eat meat. My dad has always been a huge supporter of eating meat as a source of protein. And it certainly helps with weightlifting, which Kyle loves. It was hard for him to carve out his own path and to feel comfortable giving up meat, in part because as the children of Primal diet expert Mark Sisson, our food choices have been informed and shaped by his broad knowledge about diet and exercise. But Kyle learned to embrace his own choice of diet, which is as clean and healthy as anyone else I know.

In addition to being strong athletically, as well as intellectually, I respect Kyle's ability to maintain healthy relationships. I've also learned from him to slow down and be intuitive about eating—to eat when hungry and to stop when I feel full. He cooks for himself and his friends, rarely drinks alcohol, and only recently began sipping an occasional cup of coffee. He moves his body and works his mind all day long, sometimes too much. At times I ask myself, "Where does he get all of this energy and motivation?" But then I realize that Kyle is simply in tune with his body.

I have had some great conversations with amazing people in my life, but rarely do I feel as nourished as I do after spending an evening talking about life with Kyle. Although he is three years younger than I, in so many ways, he feels older. He is my best friend. I am fortunate to have a brother whose friendship and example both nourish and inspire me.

Sweet Potato Fries

INGREDIENTS

3 sweet potatoes

Drizzle of grape seed or coconut oil

Small spoonful of garlic powder

Few pinches of salt

Drizzle of olive oil

METHOD

Preheat the oven to 400 degrees Fahrenheit. Cut three unpeeled sweet potatoes into long French-fry shapes or wedges. Drizzle grape seed or coconut oil and sprinkle a spoonful of garlic powder over the potato wedges, tossing them to cover completely. Arrange them on a cooking sheet or roasting tray, making sure to leave room between each wedge so they don't steam and soften during cooking.

Cook the potatoes for about 30 minutes, and then check them. Flip them over if you see fit and turn up the oven heat to 420 degrees Fahrenheit to cook for another 10-15 minutes or until crispy. When done and removed from the oven, drizzle a tiny bit of olive oil over the fries and salt to your liking. Toss them again, waiting a few minutes until they have cooled to enjoy!

Enjoy with dipping sauces of your choice!

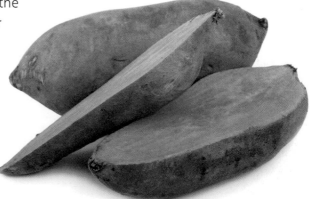

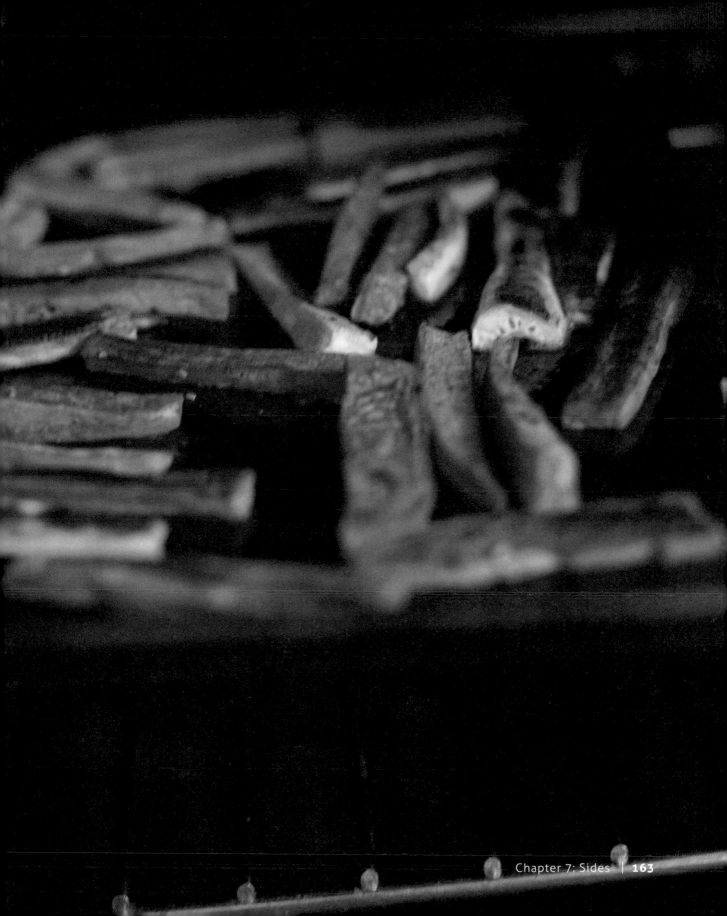

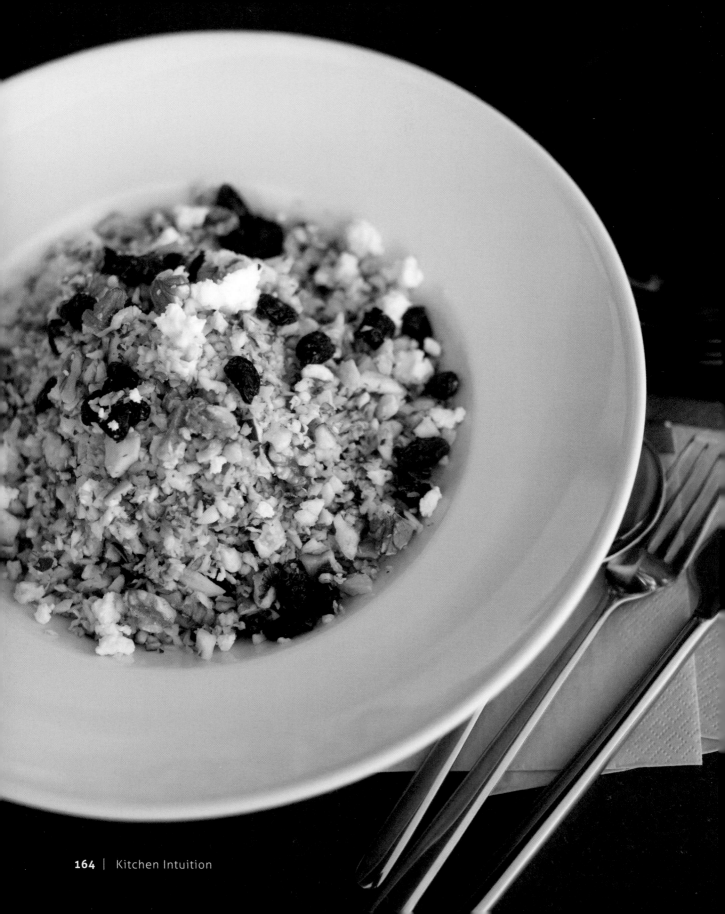

Zucchini Rice

I love this side dish because it's an entirely new way to enjoy zucchini! The crunchiness of the zucchini and walnuts go so nicely with the burst of flavor from the raisins that soak up the dressing and that tang of the smooth creamy goat cheese. Sometimes I make this with salmon, but it is delicious without as well. I always make extra so I can eat it for several days, and I'm always sad when I run out.

INGREDIENTS

2 green zucchini

Large handful of walnuts

Small handful of raisins (preferably golden)

1 dollop of mustard

A few splashes of apple cider vinegar

Small handful of goat cheese

Optional: drizzle of honey, salt, pepper, and herbs to taste

Substitutions

walnuts – pine nuts, slivered almonds

raisins – dried cherries, dried apricots, dried cranberries

METHOD

Chop the zucchini into large chunks and put them into a food processor. Pulse the processor a few times until the zucchini is the size of rice grains, then pour it into a bowl for mixing. Add a handful of lightly chopped walnuts and a handful of raisins.

In a separate bowl, whisk together a large dollop of mustard (a mustard thicker than the average watery, yellow mustard) and a few small splashes of apple cider vinegar. Whisk until the ingredients are the consistency you prefer for dressings. (Sometimes I put a tiny bit of honey in here for some sweetness.) Pour the dressing over the zucchini, walnut, and raisin mixture and toss everything together. Use your fingers to break off little bits of goat cheese (or any crumbly cheese you like) and sprinkle them over the top. Mix together one more time and give it a taste. Add any salt, pepper, herbs, or spices that you think will punch up the flavor.

Cauliflower Rosemary Mash

I love mashed potatoes, but cauliflower is much more nutrient dense and interesting in flavor. Potatoes are good, but I rarely eat one by itself (without a ton of butter and cream). Cauliflower switches it up!

INGREDIENTS

A few cups of plain, unsweetened nut milk (almond, cashew, or macadamia)

1 head of cauliflower

A few sprigs of rosemary (or a pinch, if dried)

Dash of salt

A few tablespoons butter

METHOD

Heat up a few cups of nut milk in a large pot on the stove. Chop the cauliflower into chunks and throw it into the nut milk along with the rosemary. Boil the cauliflower until it is fork tender. Then scoop and strain the cauliflower out of the pan with a slotted spoon. Strain the rosemary sprigs from the nut milk, and set the milk aside to use later.

Put the cauliflower in a blender or food processor with a dash of salt, a couple tablespoons of butter (or to taste), and a few spoonfuls of the nut milk. Blend until smooth, slowly adding more nut milk for the "mashed potato" consistency you prefer.

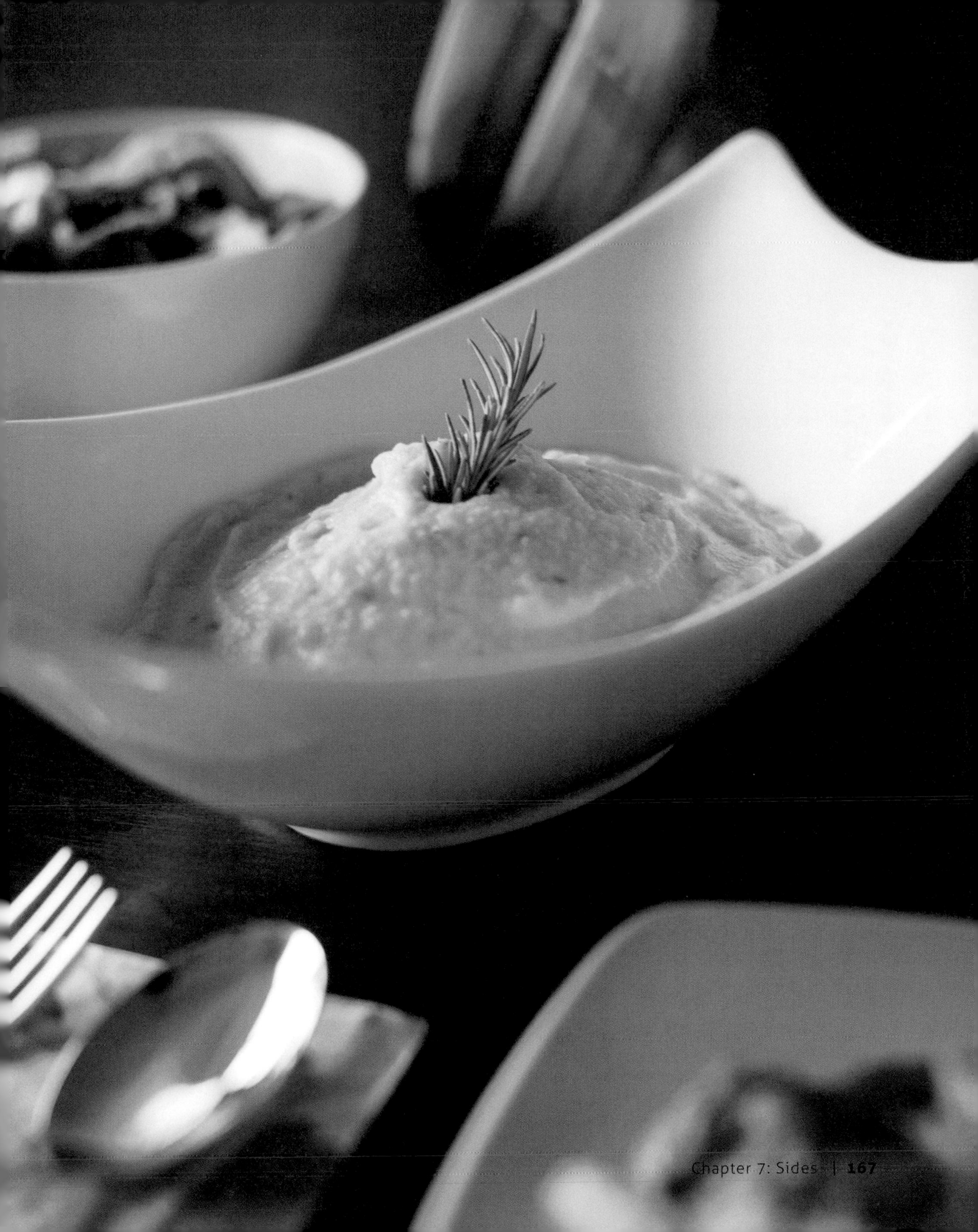

Butternut Squash

As you might be able to tell, this dish was fall-inspired. It is a beautiful side dish for Thanksgiving, but also one that I make at least once a week during the autumn and winter months. Coconut oil isn't a MUST for roasting the squash, but it lends a nice flavor and makes the house smell amazing!

INGREDIENTS

1 butternut squash

Coconut oil (to lightly coat the baking tray and squash)

Dashes of salt and pepper

A few dashes of cinnamon

Handful of feta cheese

Handful of dried cranberries

Small handful of cilantro leaves, chopped (no stems)

Optional: toasted hazelnuts

Substitutions

feta – goat cheese

dried cranberries – pomegranate seeds

cilantro – parsley

METHOD

Preheat your oven to 375 to 400 degrees Fahrenheit (depending on how hot it cooks).

Peel and cube a butternut squash. (Or, you can buy it already cubed which is much easier.) Coat a baking tray with coconut oil. Toss the cubed squash in the oil and add salt, pepper, and cinnamon.

Roast the squash for about 45 minutes, checking on it occasionally, until it is fork tender and even crispy in places. When the squash is done, add it to a bowl with a handful of crumbled cheese and the chopped herbs, dried fruit, and nuts. Mix all the ingredients together and give it a taste. What else does it need? Adjust and enjoy.

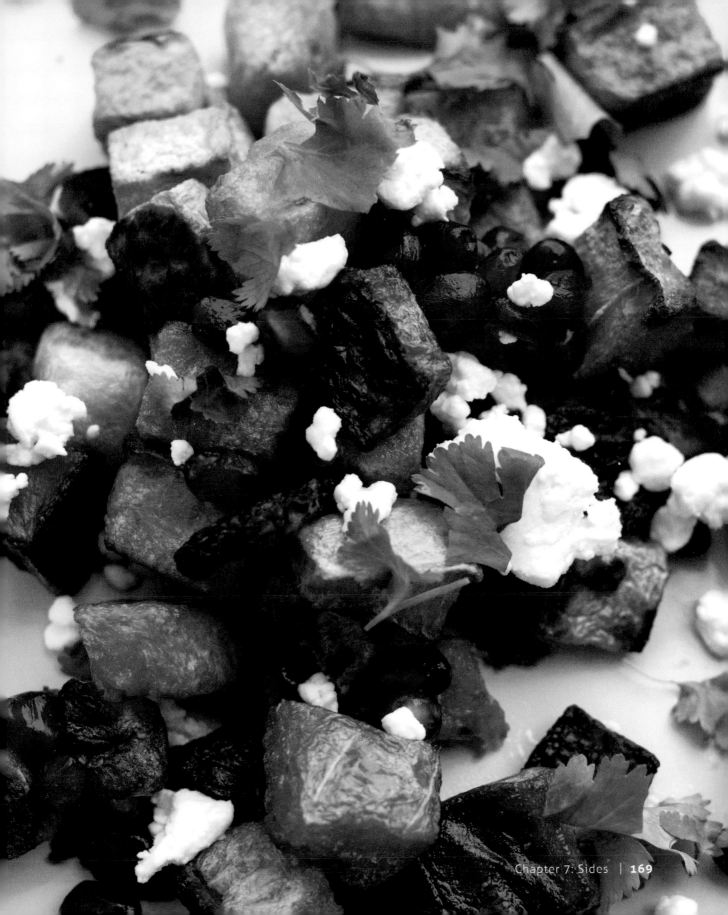

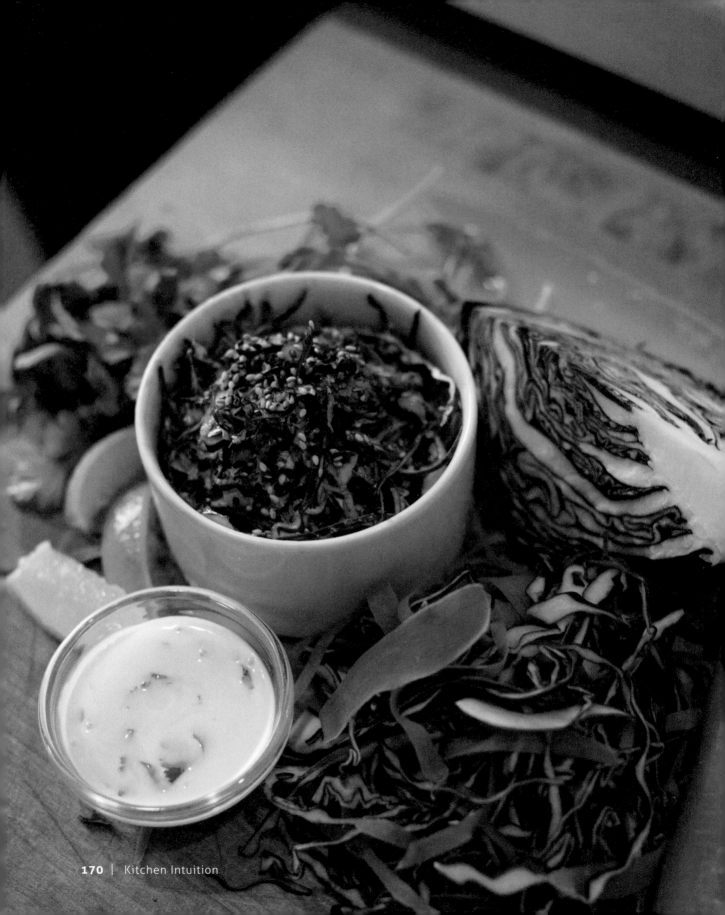

Asian Slaw

I love coleslaw. It's the go-to side dish at any BBQ restaurant I might find myself in. I decided to make my own version!

INGREDIENTS

1 red or green cabbage

Couple of carrots

2 limes, juiced

A few spoonfuls of sesame oil

1 tablespoon mayonnaise

A few sprigs of cilantro leaves, chopped

Optional: sesame seeds

METHOD

Finely shred the cabbage by either chopping it as thinly as you can or pulsing in a food processor. (You can use the largest holes on a cheese grater as a cheat.) Peel and grate the carrots.

DRESSING

Mix the juice of 2 limes, a few spoonfuls of sesame oil, and a spoonful of mayo in a small bowl. Pour the dressing over the cabbage and carrot slaw, adding chopped cilantro leaves. I top this with sesame seeds, too!

TASTE TIP

It's delicious right away, but even better the next day!

Balsamic Portabella Mushrooms

All over the food blogs, I see people talking about "meatless Monday." I don't care much for meatless Monday because I love my meat and I eat plenty of vegetables. But if one WERE to subscribe to this "meatless Monday" fad, then portabella mushrooms are a wonderful meaty alternative. Mushrooms are so healthy for you and have such a nice, thick texture that you won't feel like you're missing out on a good, square meal.

INGREDIENTS

Several portabella mushrooms
(or any mushroom of your choosing)

Couple tablespoons of olive oil

Dash of balsamic vinegar

1 to 2 tablespoons soy sauce

Dash garlic powder (or a chopped fresh garlic clove)

Coconut or olive oil, for cooking

METHOD

Slice the mushrooms into thick slices (so that when laid on their side, they look like mustaches). Place them in a Ziploc bag with olive oil, a dash of balsamic vinegar, a few squirts of soy sauce, and a chopped garlic clove (or garlic powder). Zip the bag and gently shake it around until the mushrooms are coated.

In a hot pan with olive or coconut oil, sauté the mushrooms until cooked, but still firm. Give them a taste and add more of whatever ingredient sounds good to you!

This recipe is just as delicious with a variety of mushrooms, as shown here.

VEGGIE RICE

Here is a list of ingredients to get you started, but you can really use any vegetables you like in this dish. The only ingredients I strongly recommend are the eggs, seaweed, and sesame seeds.

INGREDIENTS

1 cup of brown rice (per person)

Drizzle of olive oil, coconut oil, or butter (for cooking)

Handful of chopped veggies (especially leftovers)

1 to 2 eggs

Dash of soy sauce

Dash of sesame oil

Handful of toasted seaweed

Small handful of sesame seeds

Optional veggies: asparagus, carrots, and broccoli

METHOD

Prepare some brown rice according to the package. Chop up whatever veggies you have in the fridge into small pieces. (Leftovers are also encouraged.) In a hot pan, with a bit of heated olive oil or butter, cook the veggies. While the veggies are cooking, crack an egg or two in the hot pan, and scramble everything together.

When the rice is finished cooking, add it to the pan with the veggies. Add a dash of soy sauce and a dash of sesame oil. Crumble some toasted seaweed and some sesame seeds into the pan, and stir everything together. Give it a taste. Does it need more soy sauce or salt? Another egg? Veggies? Trust your intuition and then enjoy!

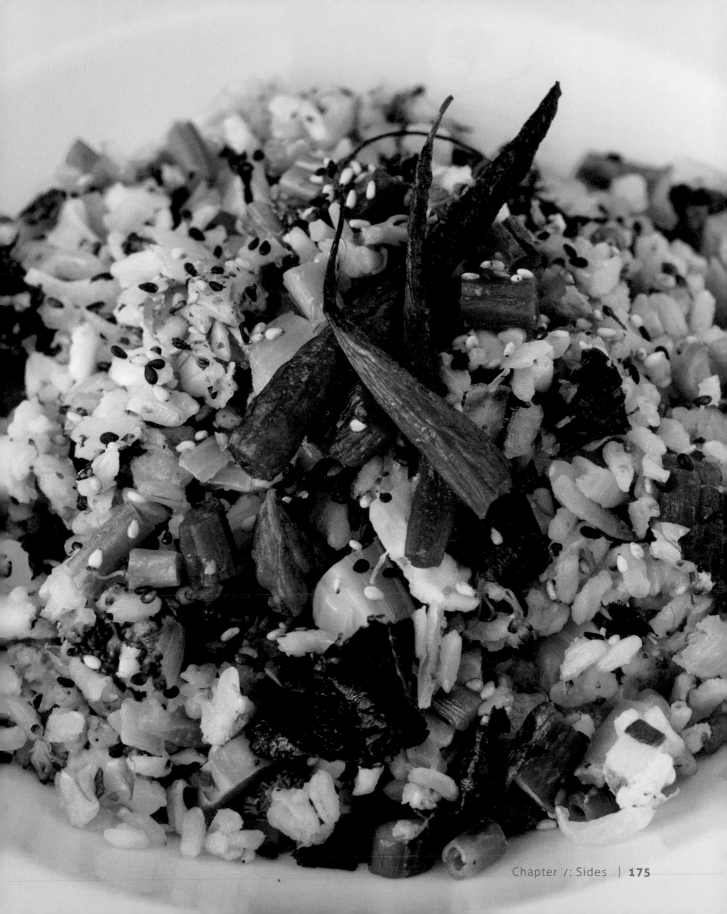

Asparagus
WITH
SUN-DRIED TOMATOES

INGREDIENTS

1 bunch of asparagus

Coconut oil or butter, for cooking

Dash of salt

Handful of pine nuts or slivered almonds

A few sun-dried tomatoes, diced

Handful of your choice of cheese

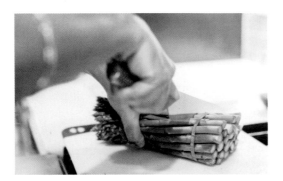

METHOD

Chop and discard the bottom inch off a bunch of washed asparagus. In a hot pan or on a grill, cook the asparagus in butter or oil until browned on each side but still crunchy. Add a dash of salt.

In a separate pan, toast some pine nuts or slivered almonds by browning them in a warm pan for a few minutes, stirring the whole time so they don't burn. When the asparagus is almost done cooking, add chopped sun-dried tomatoes and the toasted nuts to the pan of asparagus. Plate the asparagus and crumble or grate some cheese over the top. Give it a try. What do you think?

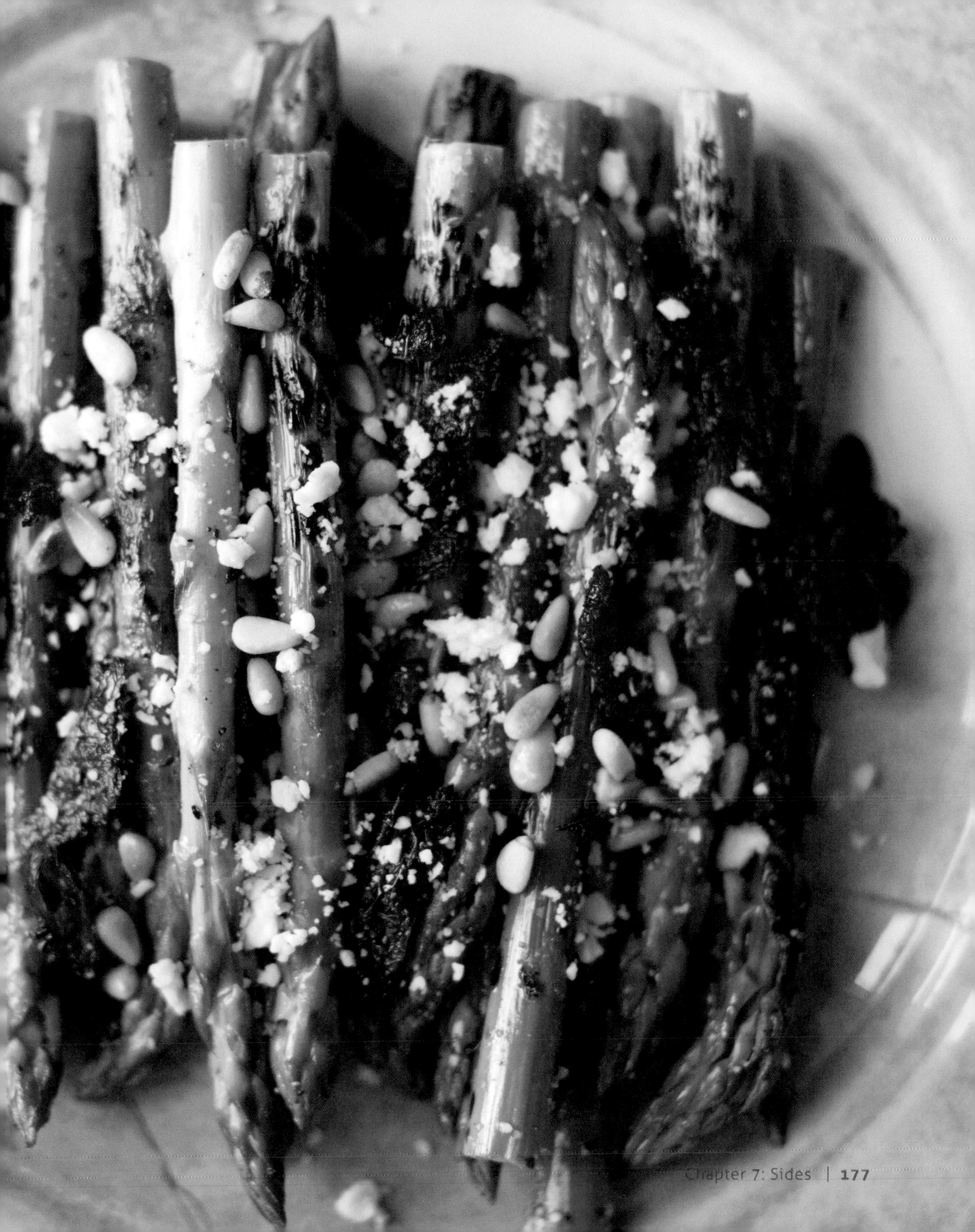

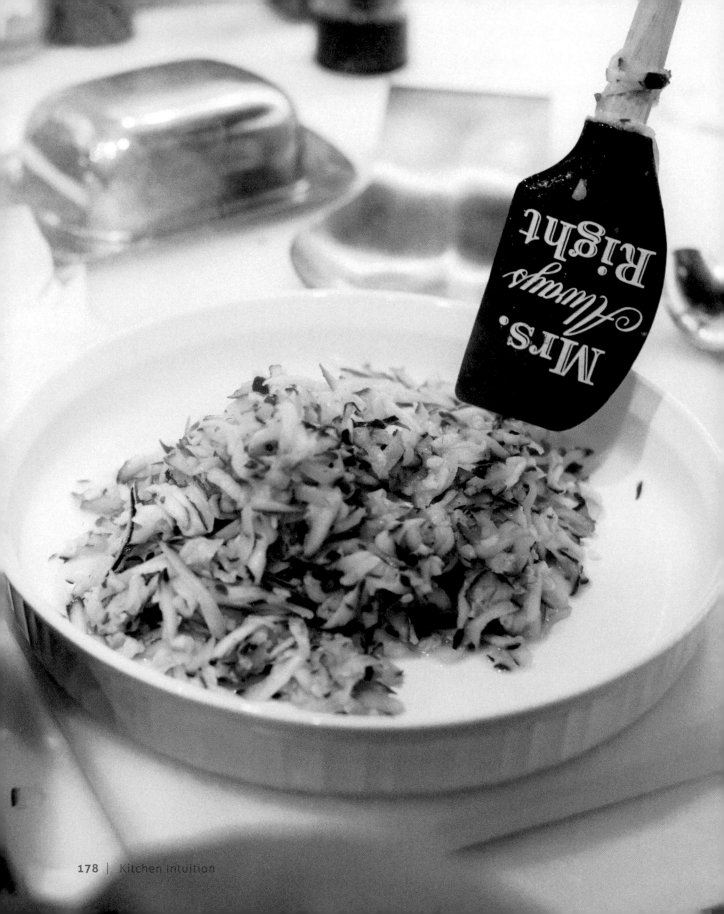

Warm Pesto Zucchini Rice

Pasta was one of my favorite things growing up. As I gain more knowledge about the world of food, I find myself not eating pasta because it has the tendency to be processed. (I would totally eat fresh pasta though!) Pesto pasta, covered in Parmesan cheese, was always one of my favorite meals. This side dish is a way for me to satisfy the pesto lover in me. It's a warm side dish with a texture that is similar to orzo (an Italian pasta that resembles rice). This goes well with grilled chicken, scallops, or salmon. But then, what doesn't go well with salmon?

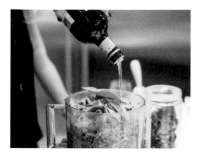 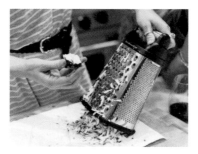 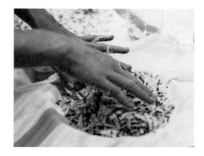

INGREDIENTS

Zucchini rice:

2 zucchini, grated

Pat of butter for cooking

Dash of salt and pepper

Pesto sauce (about 2 cups):

3 to 4 cups fresh basil (leaves only, no stems)

2 garlic cloves

¼ cup pine nuts

½ cup olive oil

½ cup Parmesan cheese

Substitutions

basil – kale (kale makes a good pesto, too)

pine nuts – walnuts, almonds

METHOD

First make the pesto sauce by blending together the basil, garlic, and pine nuts. Slowly drizzle in the olive oil. Finally, blend in the Parmesan cheese.

Grate the zucchini on the large side of a cheese grater onto a paper towel or cloth (to squeeze out excess liquid). Or you can cube the zucchini and use a food processor to pulse it into tiny pieces. Squeeze out the extra liquid. In a pan heated with butter on medium-high, stir the zucchini until heated through, adding a dash of salt and pepper to taste. Add the pesto. Taste, adjust and enjoy!

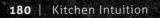

Simple Stir

This veggie stir is a staple in my home. (I call it a "stir" because I don't like the word "fry.") It's a warm, salty, and crunchy side dish that goes well with meat or fish. Simple Stir is great for days after you make it, and you can vary the veggies to eat more seasonally.

INGREDIENTS

1 red, white, or yellow onion

Handful of baby carrots or
a few regular-size carrots

1 to 2 tablespoons sesame oil

1 head of broccoli (or broccolini)

Handful of mushrooms

1 to 2 tablespoons soy sauce

2 gloves garlic

Pinch of salt

Optional: ginger (to taste; start small)

Substitutions

*You can use any vegetables you prefer;
I just like these colors and textures.*

METHOD

Cut up an onion and a few carrots (or a handful of baby carrots) into large chunks. Heat up a large pan and add 1 to 2 tablespoons of sesame oil. Throw the chopped onion and carrots into the pan first because they take the longest to cook. Add a pinch of salt—you want to flavor each layer of this dish.

While the carrots and onions are cooking, cut up a head of broccoli into bite-size pieces and slice the mushrooms. Once the carrots and onions have softened a little (give them a taste), throw in the broccoli and drizzle some soy sauce in the pan. The soy sauce adds flavor and helps the broccoli steam so that it cooks more evenly. Cover the pan for a few minutes.

When the broccoli is still crunchy but not fully cooked, add the mushrooms. If you are a garlic lover like me, chop up some garlic or even ginger and throw it in with all the ingredients right before the veggies are done cooking. (You don't want to cook the garlic for too long because it becomes bitter.) Sauté for a few more minutes until the veggies are cooked to your liking. Toss it all around and serve!

TASTE TIP

Sometimes I top this stir with a little more sesame oil and another drizzle of soy sauce.

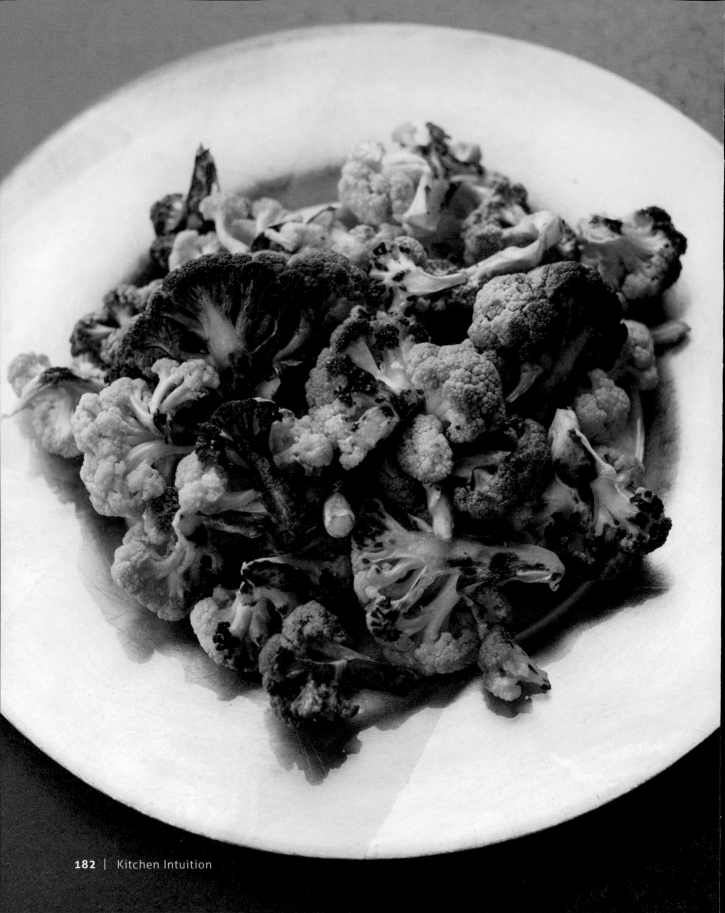

Cauliflower and Capers

I love the taste and texture of cauliflower—the crunch and nutty flavor of it. It's so pretty when grilled or roasted, and the florets are so cool looking.

INGREDIENTS

1 head of cauliflower

1 to 2 shallots

A few tablespoons of olive oil

1 to 2 lemons, juiced

Sprinkle of salt

Handful of capers

METHOD

You can cook this in a hot pan or roast in a 375-degree Fahrenheit oven. (I prefer roasting.) While the oven is preheating, chop up a head of cauliflower. (If you'd like, you can use your hands to help break up the florets into bite-size pieces.) Chop up one or two shallots. Toss the cauliflower in a bowl with olive oil, the lemon juice, and a sprinkle of salt; then spread out the cauliflower on a baking sheet. Roast in the oven for about 30 minutes (stirring occasionally) or until the cauliflower is done to your liking! Half way through cooking, take out the pan and mix in the capers and shallots with the cauliflower. Resume cooking. You may want to try another squeeze of lemon when you take it out of the oven, but let your intuition guide you.

This is great as a side dish or an afternoon snack. It keeps well in the fridge for a few days and tastes good cold or warm. You can add it to a stir-fry, some rice, or a salad later in the week. Delish!

Stuffed Mushrooms

INGREDIENTS

12 button or baby bella mushrooms

Drizzle of olive oil or pat of butter

½ onion, diced

1 to 2 garlic cloves, diced

4 cups spinach or kale, finely chopped

¼ cup pine nuts

Small handful Parmesan cheese
(or any cheese you like)

Optional: marinara sauce or pesto,
for dipping

METHOD

Preheat the oven to 350 degrees Fahrenheit. Wash the mushrooms and cut off the stems. (Set aside the stems for the stuffing.) Lightly brush the caps with olive oil, and arrange them on a baking sheet. Dice the mushroom stems pretty small. (Remember, they will have to fit into the tiny mushroom caps.) Dice both the garlic and the onions.

In a heated pan, use butter or oil to sauté the onions for a few minutes. Add the spinach (or kale) to the pan and stir until cooked. Add in the garlic, diced mushroom stems, and pine nuts to the mixture. After the sautéed mixture, has cooled enough to handle, fill the mushroom caps on the baking sheet with the mixture and top them with Parmesan cheese. Bake the stuffed mushrooms in the oven for about 30 minutes or until they are the texture you like. (Test with a fork.)

TASTE TIP

I love dipping these in marinara sauce or even some of my homemade pesto!

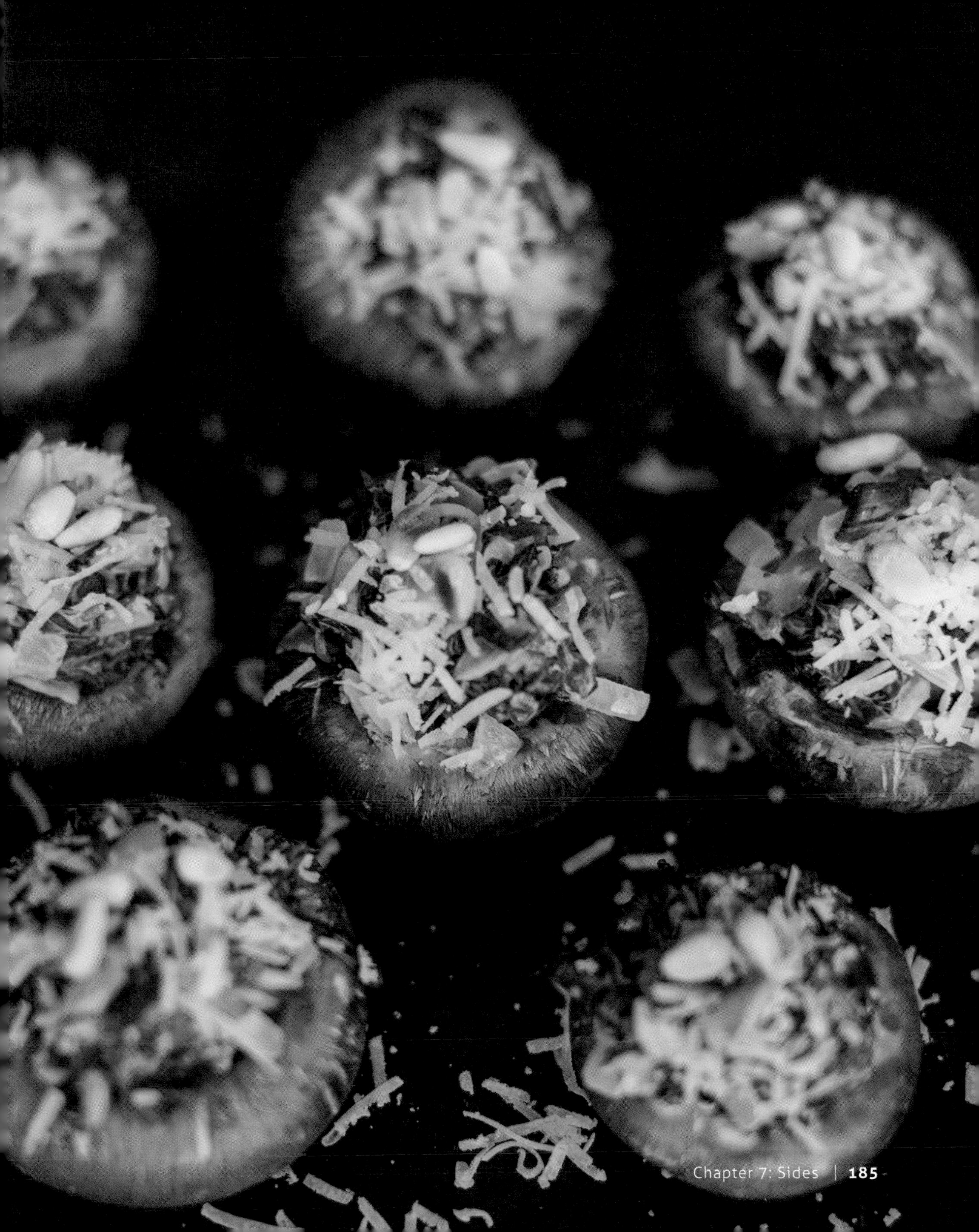

Sweet Potato Pad Thai

Get out your vegetable spiralizer—great for "zoodling" or slicing vegetables into noodle strips and shapes.

INGREDIENTS

½ to 1 sweet potato (per person)

A few spoonfuls of almond butter

2 to 3 garlic cloves

1 tablespoon/squirt sesame oil

1 to 2 limes, juiced

1 to 2 tablespoons soy sauce

1 to 2 tablespoons coconut oil, for cooking

Cilantro (as garnish)

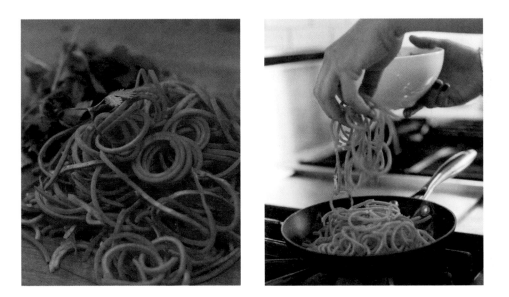

METHOD

Peel the sweet potatoes and cut off the ends before "zoodling" them into noodles with a vegetable spiralizer. In a food processor or blender, combine the almond butter, garlic cloves, sesame oil, and lime juice—blending until smooth. (If too thick, add more sesame oil, lime juice, or soy sauce, or even water, depending on your taste preference).

In a hot pan with coconut oil, cook the sweet potato "noodles" for a few minutes, adding it in one handful at a time. Just before they are done, drizzle some of the almond butter/garlic sauce over the top of the "noodles" and mix together. Garnish with some cilantro and an extra squeeze of lime!

This is everyone's favorite side dish for Thanksgiving and Christmas at our house. I am humbly in charge of making sure this dish goes according to plan (or according to intuition). I have never heard any complaints, and often I find myself stealing the leftovers from my parents' house.

INGREDIENTS

Several sweet potatoes

½ tablespoon coconut oil

Handful of pecans (or walnuts)

¼ to ½ cup maple syrup

Dash of cinnamon (and nutmeg, ginger, and allspice if you have them)

1 to 2 tablespoons butter

Pinch of salt

½ cup of almond milk (or to taste and texture you like)

METHOD

Preheat the oven to 375 degrees Fahrenheit. Poke holes in the sweet potatoes with a fork, and rub them with coconut oil. Wrap the sweet potatoes in tinfoil and bake them until super-soft, which depending on their size should be about 50 to 60 minutes.

While the potatoes are cooking, chop the nuts and place them in a hot pan on the stove. Drizzle some maple syrup over the nuts, and add the spices. Stir the nut/syrup/spice mixture around in the pan for a few minutes, as it bubbles gently. Before it gets sticky, remove from heat and set aside the mixture on a greased plate to cool. *

Once the potatoes are done (and have cooled enough to handle), peel off the skin and put them in a bowl. Add some butter, a pinch of salt, a little bit of almond milk, and mash it all together. Transfer the mashed potatoes to a casserole dish and top them with the crumbled nuts.

COOKING TIP

Make a greased plate by covering it with tinfoil and spraying or spreading butter or oil on the foil. The pecans get really sticky, so they need to cool on a surface they won't stick to.

TASTE TIP

Sometimes I put this back into the oven to warm up everything and crisp the nuts a little more, but it is good either way!

Sweet Potato Mash

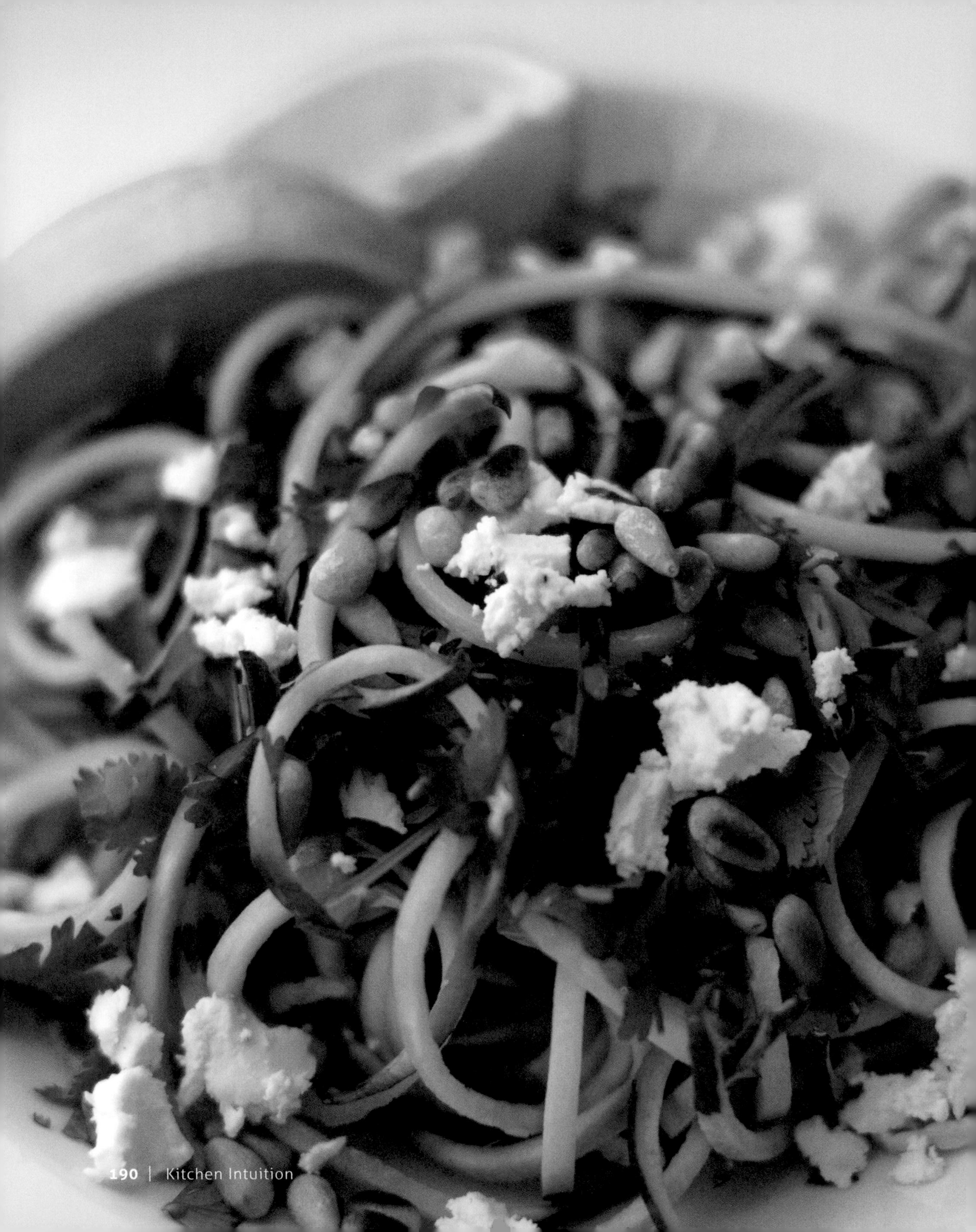

Zucchini Noodles with Lemon Herbs and Cheese

This recipe requires a "zoodler" (or a gadget that makes noodles out of veggies). They used to be big and awkward and expensive, but I found a cheap little handheld one online and it has changed my life. I highly recommend investing in one because it makes veggies even MORE fun to make.

INGREDIENTS

A few zucchini (1 per person)

1 to 2 tablespoons olive oil or butter

Sprinkle of goat or Parmesan cheese

Small handful of pine nuts

Small handful of cilantro, mint, and/or parsley, chopped (if fresh)

Squeeze of lemon

Pinch of salt

METHOD

Zoodle a few zucchini (about 1 per person), and set them aside on a paper towel. In a hot pan, drizzle some oil (or butter) and cook the zucchini noodles for 1 or 2 minutes, just until they slightly soften. Place them in a bowl and sprinkle some cheese, pine nuts, chopped herbs, a squeeze of lemon, and a pinch of salt.

TASTE TIP

This is wonderful as a pasta substitute, a delicious side dish, or as a bed for a nice piece of chicken or salmon.

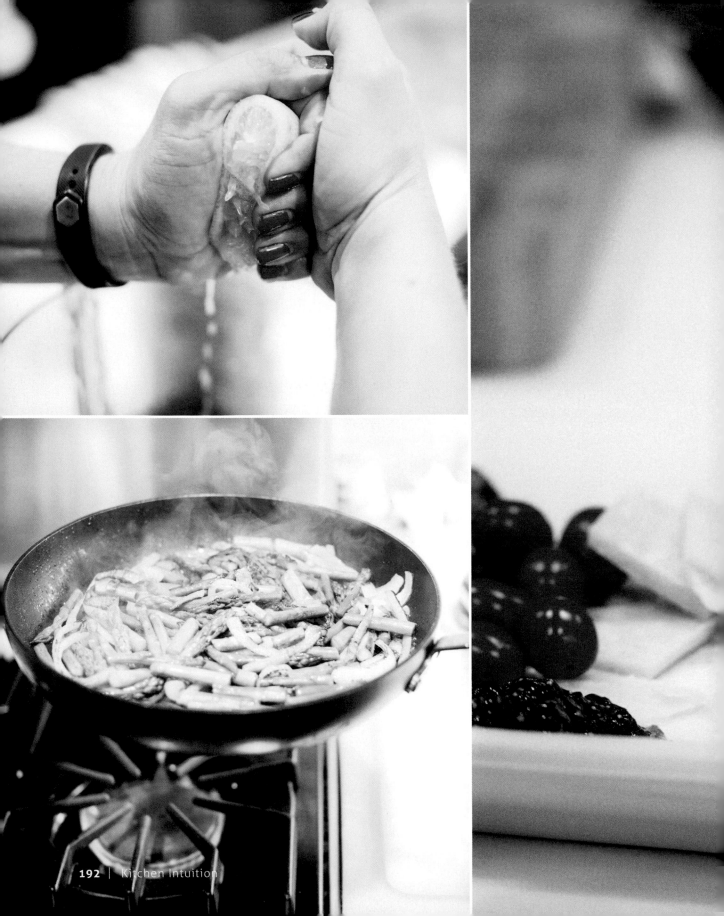

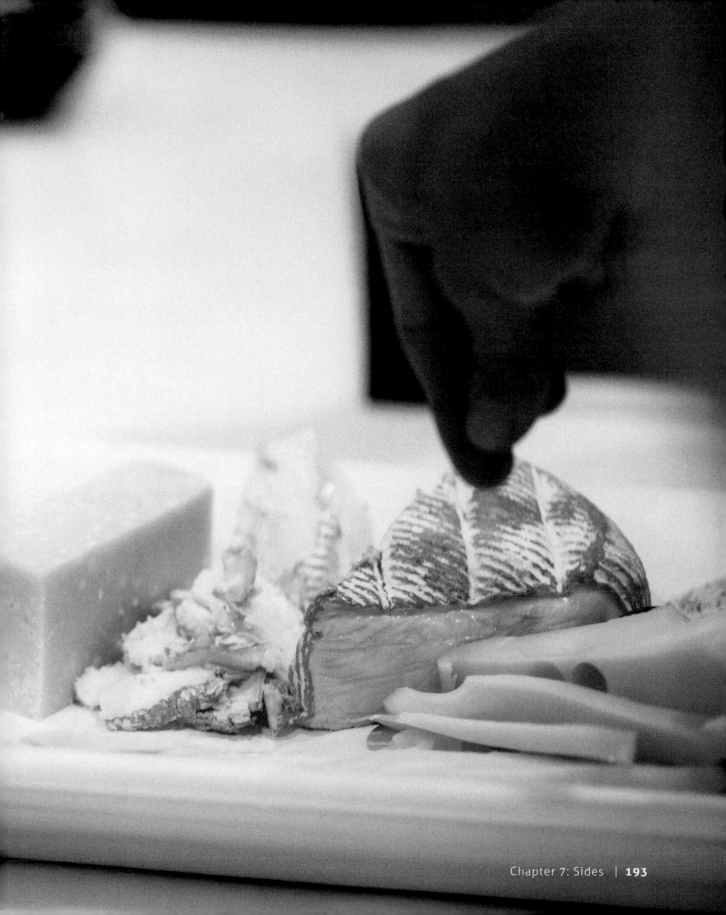

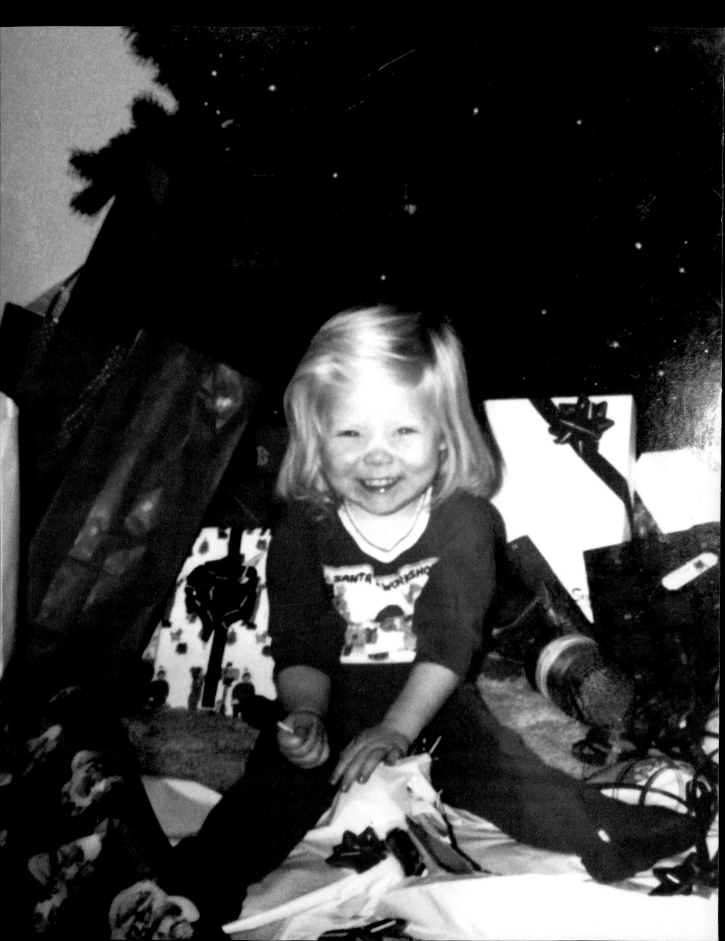

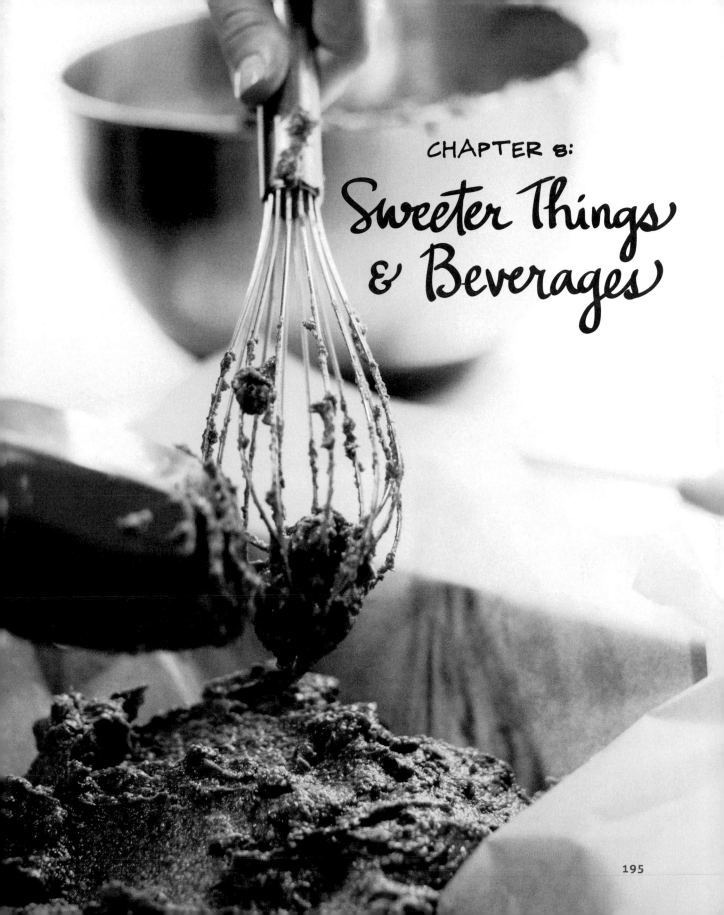

CHAPTER 8:

Sweeter Things & Beverages

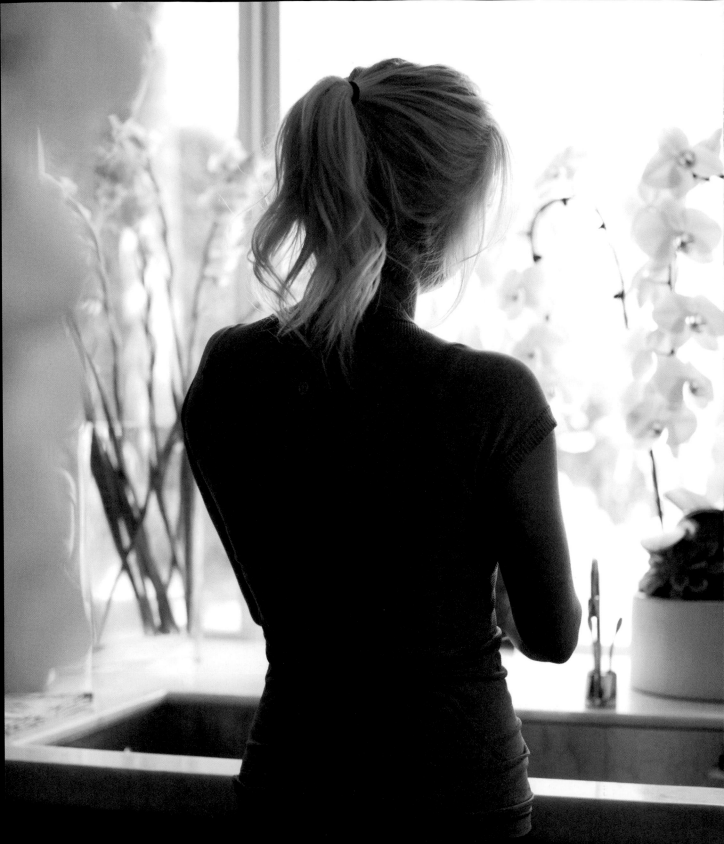

Kitchen Story: If I'm Being Honest

If I'm being real with you, writing this book hasn't been easy, and no published author will tell you their first draft of ANY book was exciting and new and fun the entire time. When I started writing this book, I would get creative spurts of energy and write for hours (the cooking part was always effortless). The hardest part was sharing my honest experience with food and my relationship to my body with you.

I can easily share with anyone who is willing to listen how to cook, how to love their body, cure their illnesses, and how to cultivate all things *intuitive*. But I hit a major roadblock when I felt like I wasn't consistently *doing* those things for myself. Struggling with my health for about a year, I felt anxious and lost, off balance, and out of touch with my intuition. I stopped writing and sharing because I felt like a fraud. *Who am I to tell YOU how to do it when I'm not even doing it myself?* This is one of the many reasons that I admire my dad; he talks the talk and walks the walk.

Just as you want your dentist to have nice teeth, your doctor to be in good health, and your trainer to be fit, shouldn't I be expected to have my stuff together before preaching to others? The answer I have come to understand is: not necessarily, because we are all human and we all struggle sometimes. If everyone had to be at their very best before we could share with each other the valuable lessons we've learned, we wouldn't get very far.

During the lengthy hiatus I took from writing, I would still talk about *Kitchen Intuition* with everyone I met as if I was actively working on it and just as excited about it as the day the idea came to mind. I even shared with people how I felt like a fraud, how I wasn't quite done because I was waiting to be in perfect shape before I finished. The feedback I got from those people is the reason I mustered up the courage to continue. People wanted to know about my setbacks because it was a reminder that it is okay to be human after all.

Their encouragement to keep writing because they felt my stories could help them or their loved ones gave me the impetus to continue. Ironically enough, in the beginning of this book I encouraged you to mess up, not to worry about burning or over-salting things or messing up a perfectly good meal, yet here I was, not allowing myself to mess up at all. Well, this cookbook is proof in the pudding that I didn't let a little self-doubt stop me. Nor, should you.

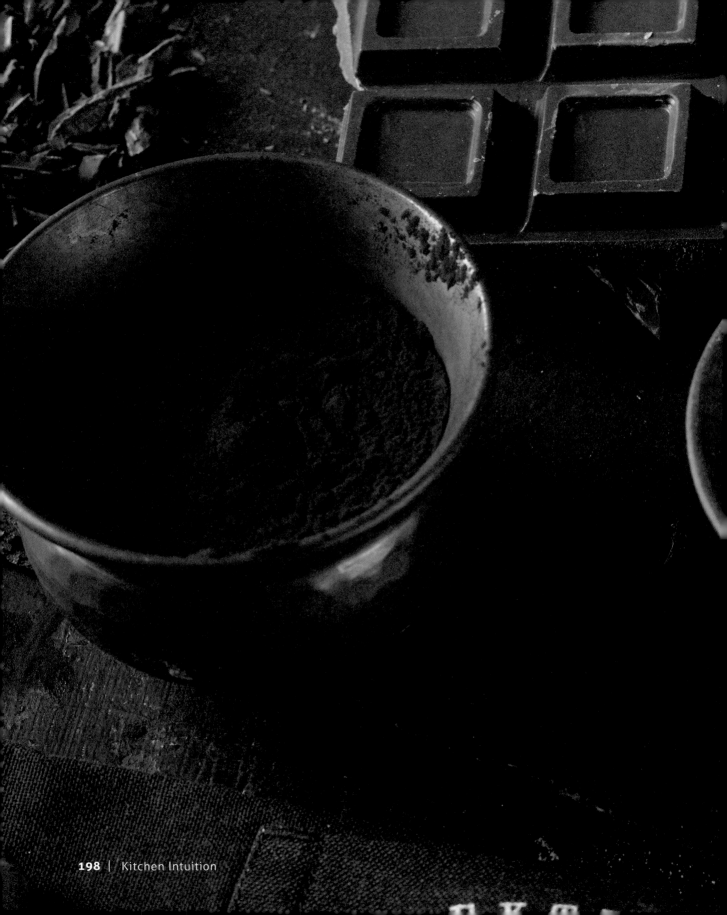

Sweeter Things

We all love our sweets, but let's face it, the more we focus on eating healthier greens and protein, the better off we feel. There are still ways to satisfy your sweet tooth and eat healthy however, and I've included some of my favorite quick fixes here. Remember, experimenting and playing with recipes is half the fun to enjoying your own sweet treat.

Chia Pudding

Chia pudding is a ratio of chia seeds to liquid, usually 1:1 or 1:2.

Making chia pudding is easy. Use the directions on the back of the package. You will probably need only water, coconut water, nut milk, or coconut milk to make it. I prefer nut milk.

Chocolate Chia Mousse

Use the same directions to make chia pudding from the above recipe and then add:

A few pieces of dark chocolate (shaved or chopped),
or a few spoonfuls of cacao powder

2 spoonfuls of maple syrup (honey or agave syrup works also)

METHOD
Blend ingredients in a Cuisinart or blender.

Taste the pudding to see if it needs more chocolate or sweetener. I like to top this one with mint leaves and cacao nibs!

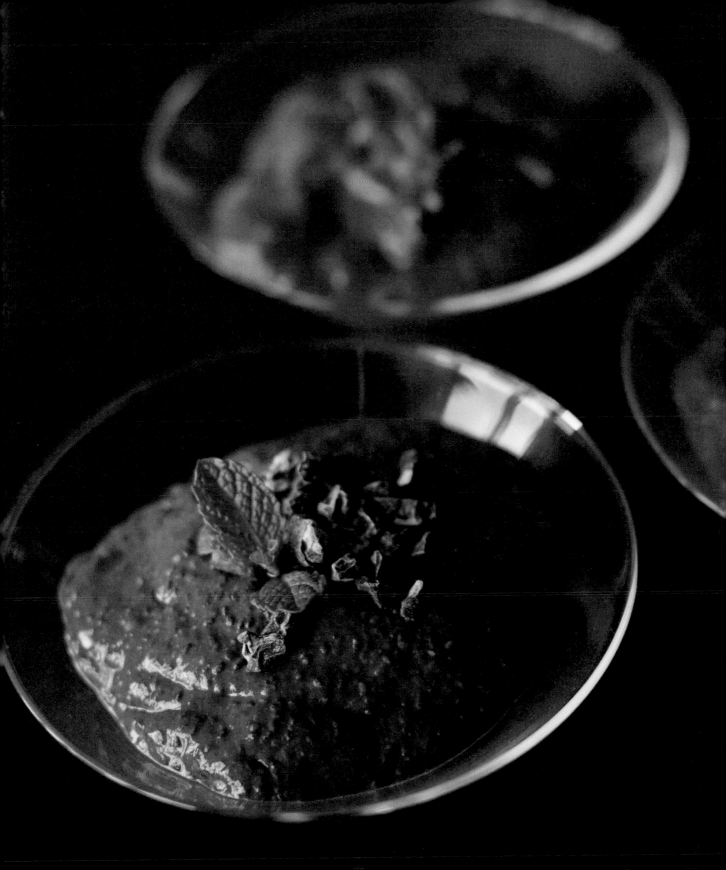

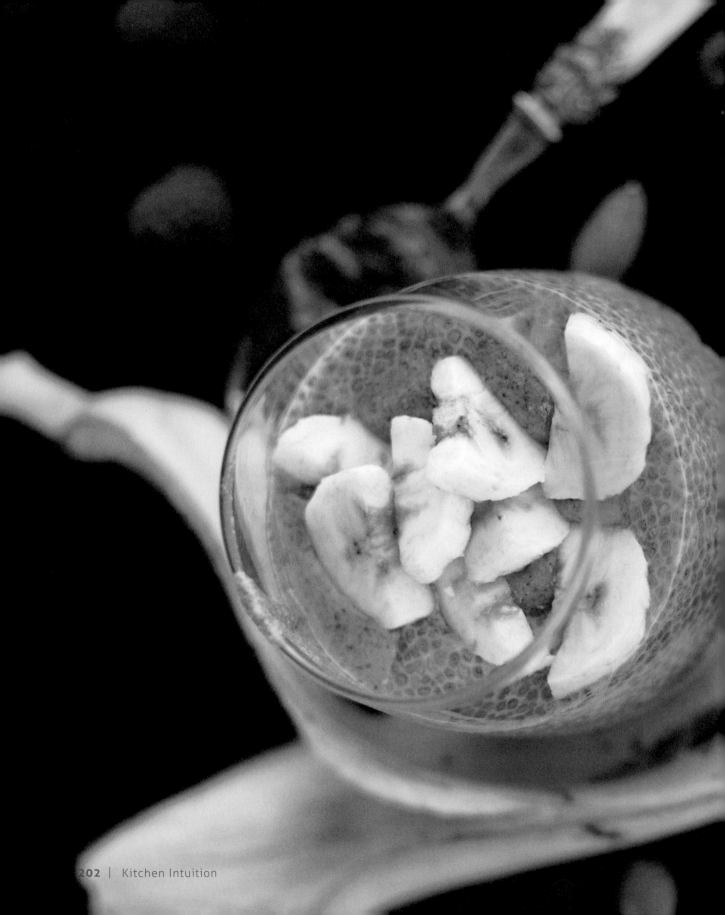

Banana and Berry Chia Parfait

After you've made the chia pudding, layer it with:

1 banana, sliced (or mushed)

Handful of berries

1 to 2 spoonfuls of almond butter (or Nutella, or peanut butter and jelly *and* berries!)

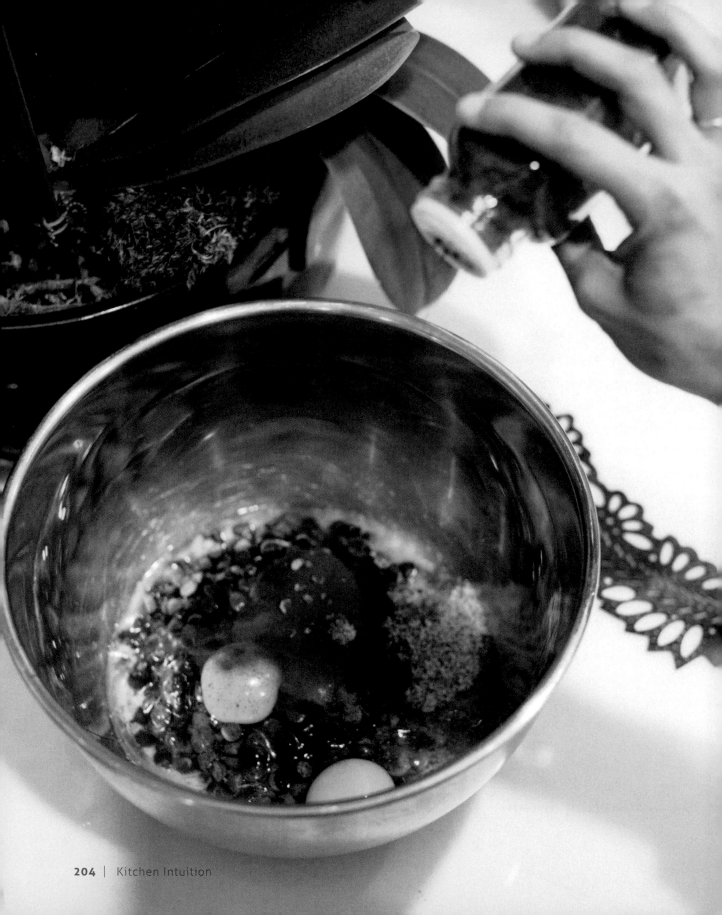

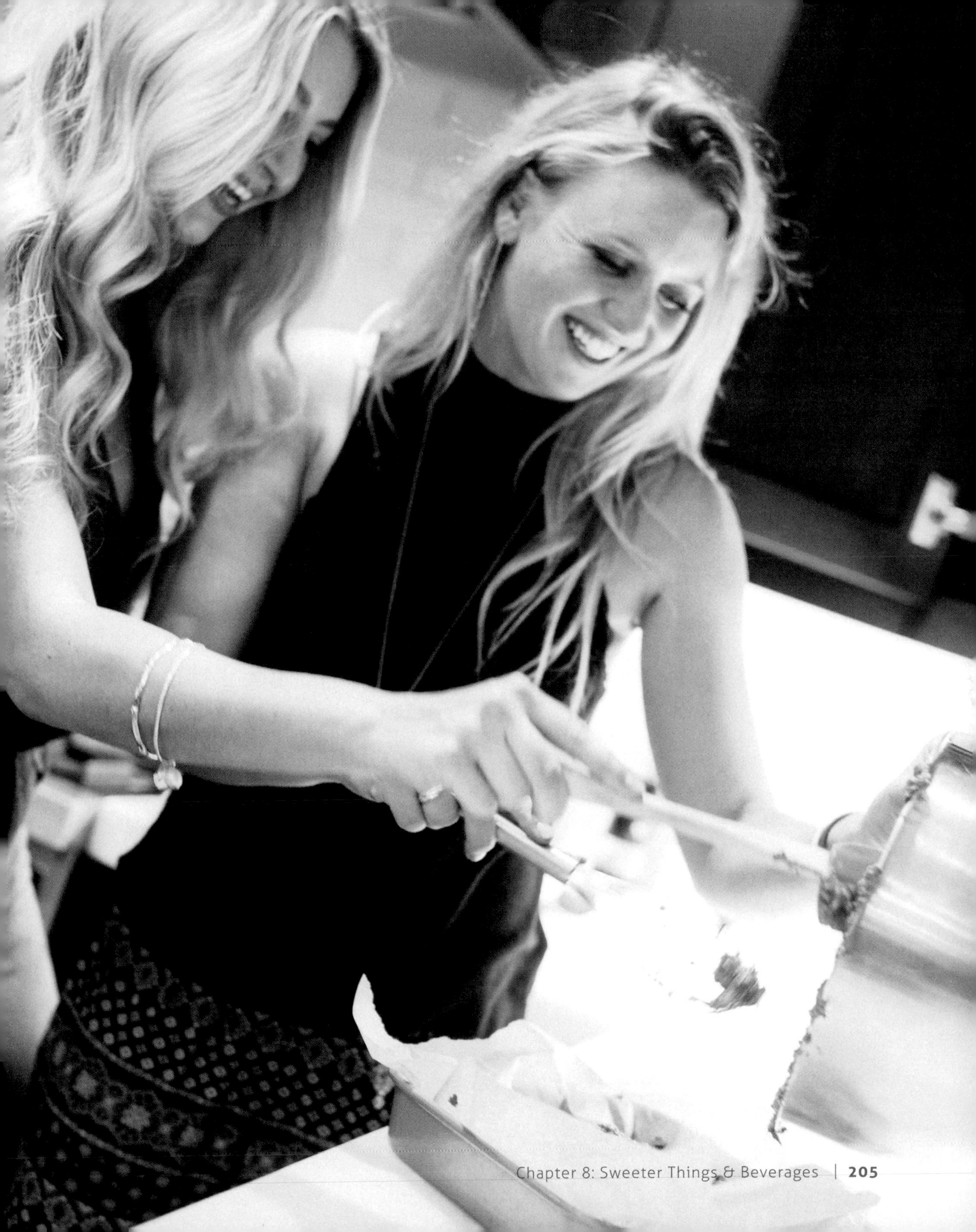

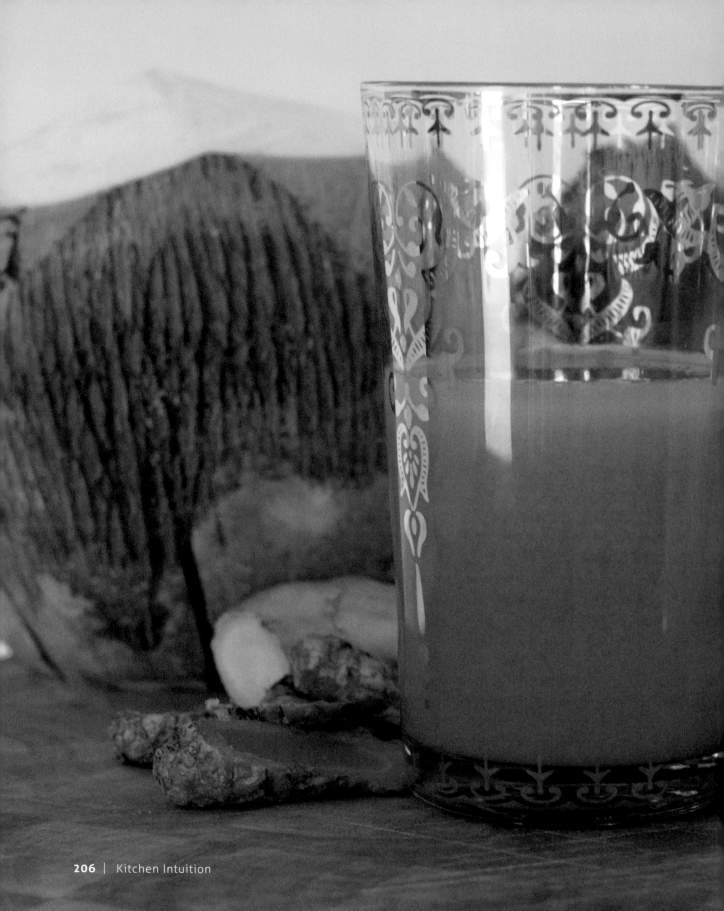

Dev's Bevs

TO HYDRATE, NOURISH, AND SOMETIMES WARM UP!

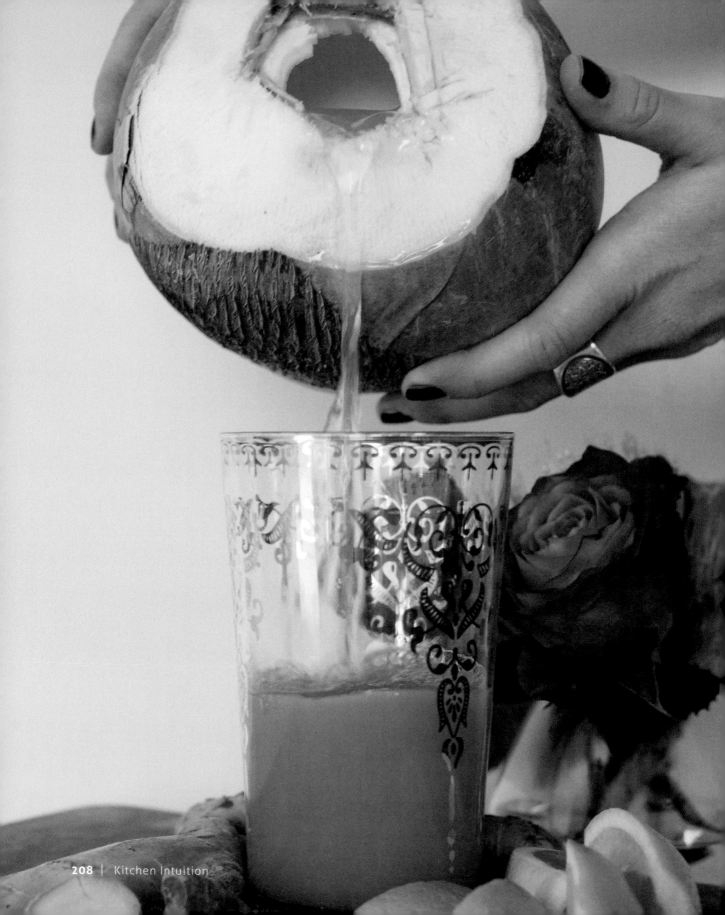

Devynade

I invented this at my local and beloved juice bar because I like the idea of wellness shots. I LOVE the taste of coconut water, so I thought "why not put all the wellness shot ingredients into there?" It tastes like ginger lemonade. And I drink it Every. Single. Day.

INGREDIENTS

1 serving of coconut water (fresh or bottled—make sure its organic)

1-ounce shot of turmeric (juiced or pressed)

1-ounce shot of ginger (juiced or pressed)

1 lemon (juiced or pressed)

METHOD

Mix all the ingredients together, drink and enjoy!

Herby Water

Drinking only water to stay hydrated feels like a chore because I don't find the "taste" of water to be that interesting. I started adding herbs and citrus in a water pitcher and then refrigerating it over night! Now I'm actually excited to hydrate with water! Plus it looks super cool.

ADD ANY OF THE FOLLOWING TO A PITCHER OF WATER:

mint leaves

basil leaves

sliced ginger

lemon slices

orange slices

lime slices

sage leaves

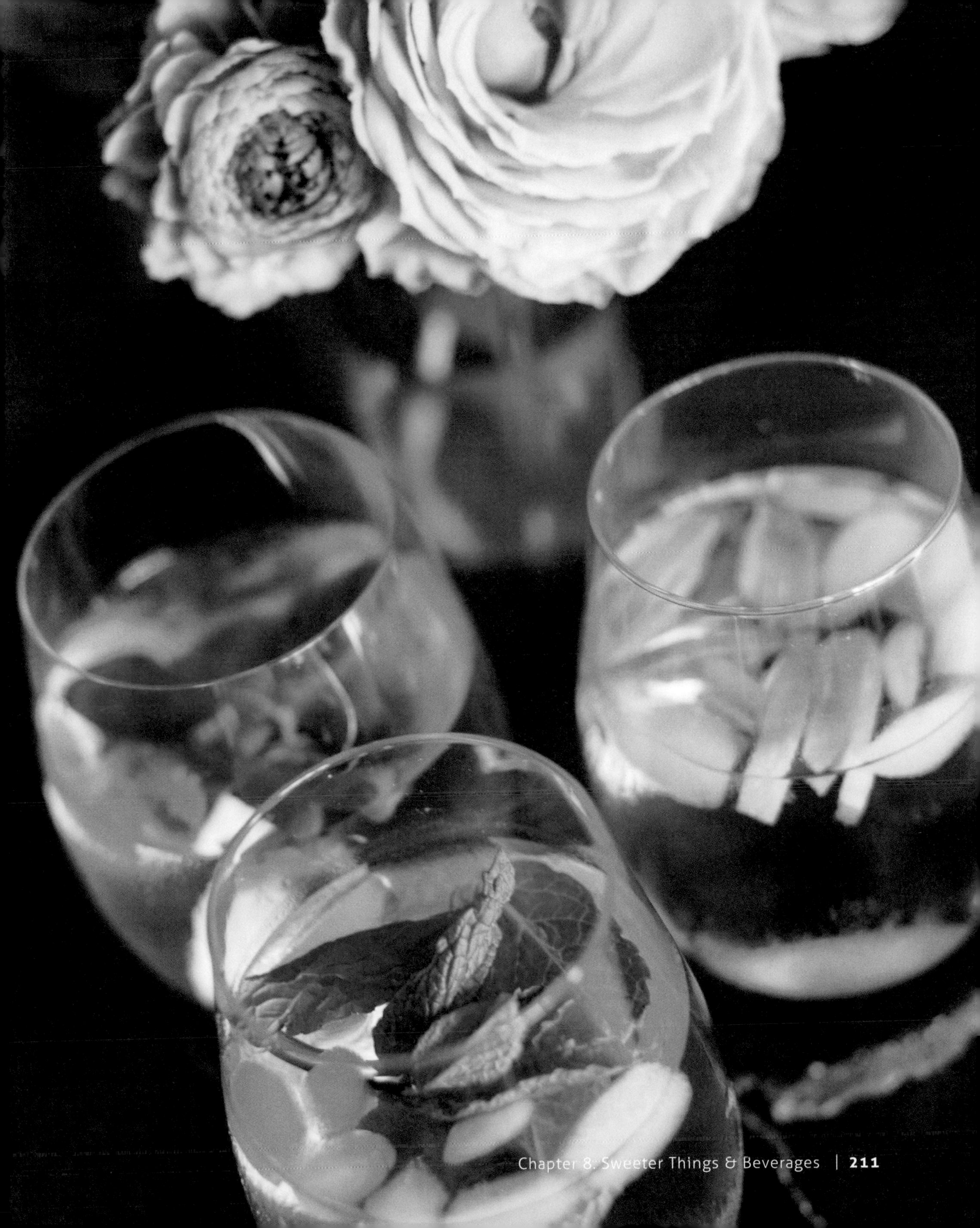

Almond (Nut) Milk

You can do this same process with most raw nuts to make delicious nut milks. I make it plain to use as the "cream" in my soups and vegetable mashes. I sweeten it to use in my smoothies or in coffee and tea. You can also freeze the "milk" in ice cube trays and add them when blending smoothies.

INGREDIENTS

Few handfuls of raw organic nuts

Few cups of water

To sweeten:

Spoon of maple syrup

Dash of cinnamon, nutmeg, or ginger

1 to 2 dates, pitted

METHOD

Soak a few handfuls of RAW almonds (or cashews, macadamia nuts, etc.) in a bowl of water overnight. A few hours will do, too.

Drain the ingredients with a strainer, and then drain a second time with cheesecloth. (I cheat and use a hand towel sometimes.)

Toss the almonds (or other nuts) into a blender with a few cups of fresh water. If you want to sweeten it for smoothies, drinks, or coffee, add a pinch of each spice, a spoon of maple syrup, and 1 or 2 dates (pitted). Blend for a few minutes. Give it a taste to see if you would like it any more sweetener or spice, and adjust accordingly.

TASTE TIP

The sweetened version of the recipe is best for smoothies, for drinking, and for coffee. If you choose to make nut milk to add to recipes, then it is best to leave the sweeteners and spices out, and instead just blend the nuts and water.

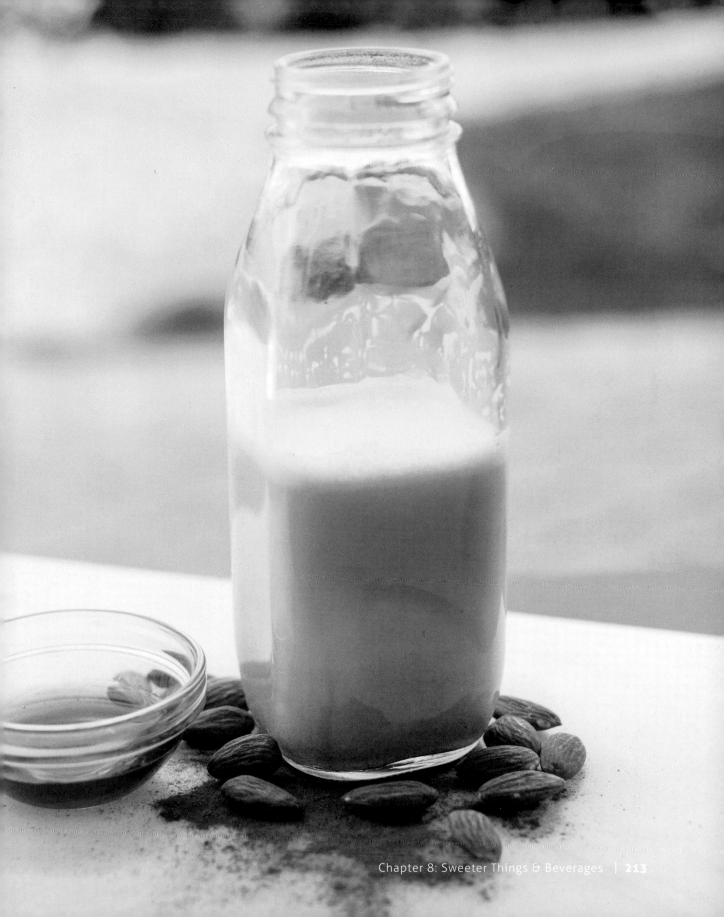

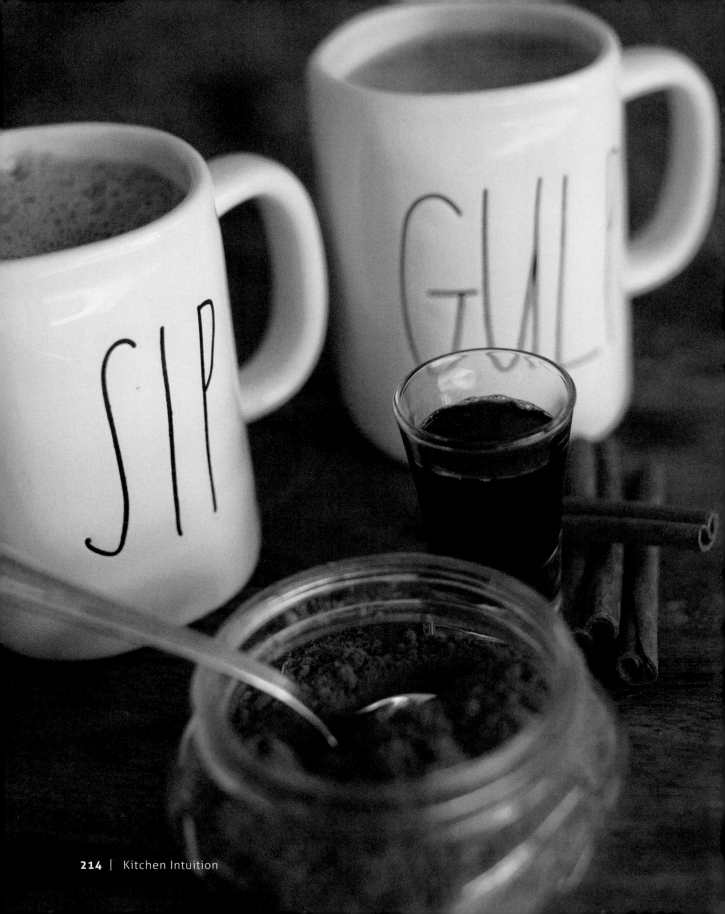

HOT Cocoa

I melt chocolate into almond milk as it warms on the stove and whisk it until it is frothy. Sometimes I add spices like cinnamon or maple syrup to give it some extra sweetness.

INGREDIENTS

1 cup almond milk

Few spoonfuls of cocoa or shaved chocolate

Optional: dash of cinnamon or spoon of maple syrup

Smoothies

Smoothies are great for breakfast and a quick snack. They are versatile because almost any fruit (and even some veggies) can be thrown into a blender with some ice and protein powder. If the smoothie comes out too thick, simply add more liquid. Adjusting the flavor is an easy fix. Just add some juice or more fruit.

ALL SMOOTHIES SERVE 1 PERSON

Blueberry Almond Butter Smoothie

Blueberry Almond Butter
S M O O T H I E

INGREDIENTS

Handful of ice cubes

Handful of frozen or fresh blueberries

½ banana

1 spoonful of almond butter

1 cup of almond milk (or any nut milk/coconut water will do)

Optional:

2 dates (to sweeten),

flaxseeds,

chia seeds,

coconut oil,

protein powder,

dried goji berries

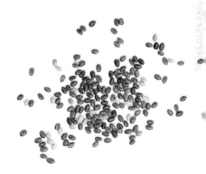

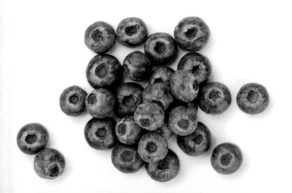

Strawberry ginger Smoothie

INGREDIENTS

Small handful of ice cubes

Handful of frozen or fresh strawberries

2 big spoonfuls of yogurt (I like Greek yogurt because it's a little sour, but any yogurt will do)

Few slices of fresh, peeled ginger

1 cup of coconut milk or coconut water

Dark Chocolate Cherry Smoothie

INGREDIENTS

Small handful of ice cubes

Big handful of frozen cherries or fresh cherries (if fresh, make sure to take out the pits!)

1 scoop of cacao powder or chocolate protein powder

2 dates, pitted

1 cup of almond milk (or any nut milk you like)

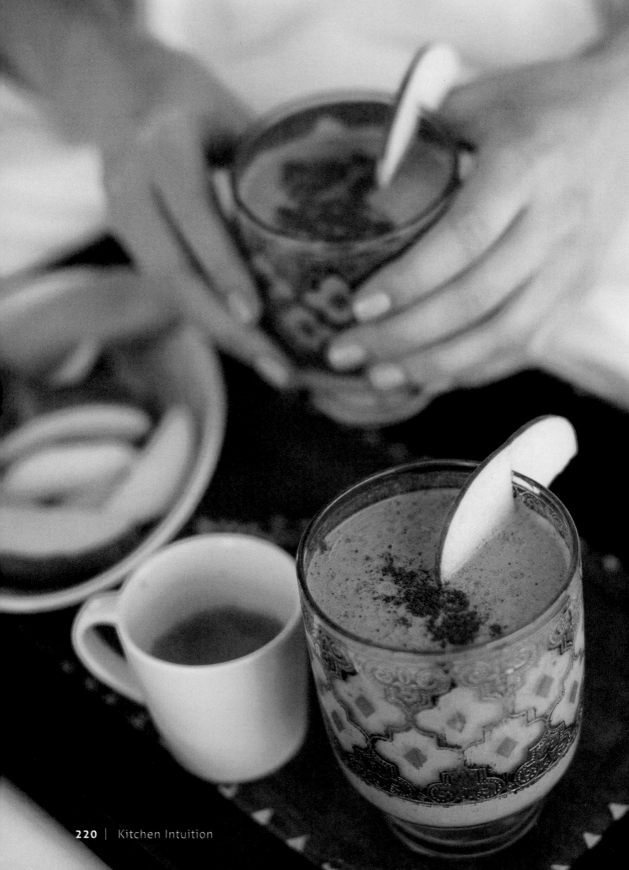

Apple Pie Smoothie

INGREDIENTS

Small handful of ice cubes

1 red or yellow/red apple, cut into chunks

Dash of cinnamon

Dash of ginger (or a piece of fresh ginger)

Dash of nutmeg

½ banana

Few spoonfuls of vanilla yogurt (or vanilla protein powder)

Handful of flax seeds or spoonful of flax seed oil

1 cup of almond milk

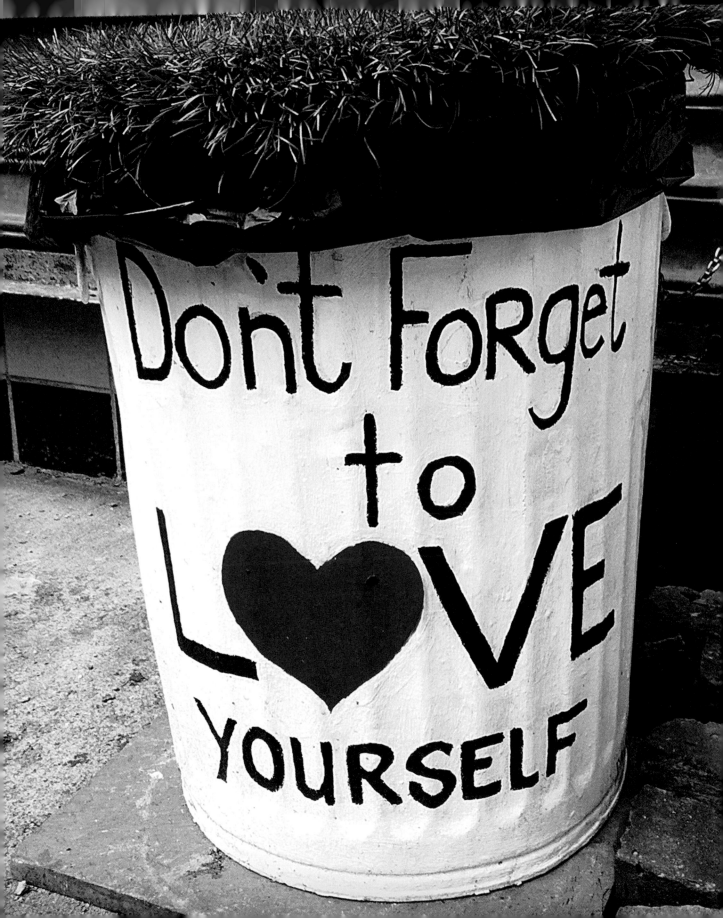

INDEX